Shed Some Pounds

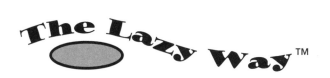

Shed Some Pounds

Annette Cain and Becky Carlson

The Lazy Way™

Macmillan • USA

To Joan—A mother, a friend, on whose love and wisdom you can depend.

Macmillan Publishing books may be purchased for business or sales promotional use. For information please write: Special Markets Department, Macmillan Publishing USA, 1633 Broadway, New York, NY 10019.

International Standard Book Number: 0-02-862999-X
Library of Congress Catalog Card Number: 98-89490

01 00 99   8 7 6 5 4 3 2 1

Interpretation of the printing code: the rightmost number of the first series of numbers is the year of the book's printing; the rightmost number of the second series of numbers is the number of the book's printing. For example, a printing code of 99-1 shows that the first printing occurred in 1999.

Printed in the United States of America

Book Design: Madhouse Studios

Page Creation by Carrie Allen, Eric Brinkman, and Heather Pope.

You Don't Have to Feel Guilty Anymore!

IT'S O.K. TO DO IT *THE LAZY WAY*!

It seems every time we turn around, we're given more responsibility, more information to absorb, more places we need to go, and more numbers, dates, and names to remember. Both our bodies and our minds are already on overload. And we know what happens next—cleaning the house, balancing the checkbook, and cooking dinner get put off until "tomorrow" and eventually fall by the wayside.

So let's be frank—we're all starting to feel a bit guilty about the dirty laundry, stacks of ATM slips, and Chinese take-out. Just thinking about tackling those terrible tasks makes you exhausted, right? If only there were an easy, effortless way to get this stuff done! (And done right!)

There is—*The Lazy Way*! By providing the pain-free way to do something—including tons of shortcuts and time-saving tips, as well as lists of all the stuff you'll ever need to get it done efficiently—*The Lazy Way* series cuts through all of the time-wasting thought processes and laborious exercises. You'll discover the secrets of those who have figured out *The Lazy Way*. You'll get things done in half the time it takes the average person—and then you will sit back and smugly consider those poor suckers who haven't discovered *The Lazy Way* yet. With *The Lazy Way,* you'll learn how to put in minimal effort and get maximum results so you can devote your attention and energy to the pleasures in life!

The Lazy Way PROMISE

Everyone on *The Lazy Way* staff promises that, if you adopt *The Lazy Way* philosophy, you'll never break a sweat, you'll barely lift a finger, you won't put strain on your brain, and you'll have plenty of time to put up your feet. We guarantee you will find that these activities are no longer hardships, since you're doing them *The Lazy Way*. We also firmly support taking breaks and encourage rewarding yourself (we even offer our suggestions in each book!). With *The Lazy Way*, the only thing you'll be overwhelmed by is all of your newfound free time!

The Lazy Way SPECIAL FEATURES

Every book in our series features the following sidebars in the margins, all designed to save you time and aggravation down the road.

- **"Quick n' Painless"**—shortcuts that get the job done fast.

- **"You'll Thank Yourself Later"**—advice that saves time down the road.

- **"A Complete Waste of Time"**—warnings that spare countless headaches and squandered hours.

- **"If You're So Inclined"**—optional tips for moments of inspired added effort.

- **"The Lazy Way"**—rewards to make the task more pleasurable.

If you've either decided to give up altogether or have taken a strong interest in the subject, you'll find information on hiring outside help with "How to Get Someone Else to Do It" as well as further reading recommendations in "If You Really Want More, Read These." In addition, there's an only-what-you-need-to-know glossary of terms and product names ("If You Don't Know What It Means/Does, Look Here") as well as "It's Time for Your Reward"—fun and relaxing ways to treat yourself for a job well done.

With *The Lazy Way* series, you'll find that getting the job done has never been so painless!

Series Editor
Amy Gordon

Managing Editor
Robert Shuman

Editorial Director
Gary Krebs

Development Editor
Alana J. Morgan

Director of Creative Services
Michele Laseau

Production Editor
Christy Wagner

Cover Designer
Michael Freeland

What's in This Book

It's a Piece of Cake!

Shedding some pounds *The Lazy Way* is a piece of cake! You won't have to follow any detailed instructions for eating. There's no beating or whipping you into exercising. And changing those bad habits can be as smooth as silk. When you follow the Lazy recipe, losing your weight couldn't get any sweeter.

This book will give you all the ingredients you need for shedding your pounds permanently.

- How to cut the fat without sacrificing taste or time.
- Tricks for portion control and tips for avoiding the spread and boosting the shed.
- How to eat healthy on the go.
- The bare minimum you need to move to get results.
- How to slip exercise into the busiest of schedules.
- Simple strengthening exercises you can do at home, at the gym, or in your chair.
- How to set goals you can achieve (finally!).
- Tricks and treats to help you think positively.
- Effortless strategies to lose the bad habits and gain alternative desirable ones.
- Clothing tips that will make you lose inches instantly.

So, get ready to devour all of the great information in this book. You can feast on it one piece at a time (chapters) or indulge yourself with little bites (sidebars). When you're done you'll savor being fit for a lifetime.

THANK YOU . . .

Bob Carlson, Greg Rhines, Jim Vaughn, Martha Casselman, Stephanie Prima Sarantopulos of The Savory Times™, family and friends, San Tomo Team, and the team at Macmillan.

Disclaimer

This book is not intended as a substitute for professional medical advice. As with all weight-loss and exercise programs, you should obtain your physician's permission, especially if you have a medical problem such as diabetes, high blood pressure, or heart disease. The authors disclaim any liability arising directly or indirectly from the use and application of any of the contents of this book.

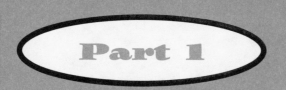

Part 1

Here's the Skinny

Are You Too Lazy to Read Here's the Skinny?

1 You spend more time weighing your food than you do eating it. ☐ yes ☐ no

2 Watching what you eat only make you feel guilty because you don't think you've attained your goals (and then you reach for the bag of chips). ☐ yes ☐ no

3 "Working out" makes you think of having to go to the gym, sweating in front of people you don't know, and worrying about not being as in shape as everyone else. ☐ yes ☐ no

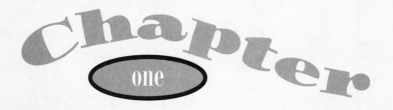
The Lard Works in Mysterious Ways

Welcome to the Land of Loss, where shedding pounds is as easy as popping some pills and clicking your heels. Oh my! This would make more than even Dorothy's dreams come true. We all want that quick fix, especially when it comes to losing weight. Even though we can't depend on magic to shrink us down, that doesn't mean you we have to follow a long, hard road. You can shed your pounds *The Lazy Way* and get results with just a little effort.

Yes, we did say effort, though the key word is "little." Everything worthwhile takes some effort, but there's no point in spinning your wheels. The key is to be smart and efficient about how you tackle what's ahead of you (and behind you too!). And that's what the lazy approach to pound shedding is all about.

In this chapter, we'll take the mystery out of how weight loss works and reveal what definitely does not work. Then, we'll give you the intimate details on what it takes as far as

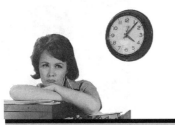

your eating, exercise, and attitude, to shed some pounds *The Lazy Way*.

WHAT STROLLS IN MUST WANDER OUT

There's no big mystery to how the body loses weight. It basically boils down to creating caloric deficits, increasing muscle mass, and decreasing fat stores.

The Almighty Deficit

We all know how to create a deficit with our bank accounts. Here's how it works with calories.

- You create a safe and healthy caloric deficit when you cut back on calories consumed and increase calories burned.

- You must be in a deficit of 3,500 calories before you can lose a pound of fat (1 pound of fat = 3,500 calories).

- If you take in more calories than you burn off, those extra calories will be stored as fat.

It Ain't Heavy, It's My Muscle

Here's why you don't want to complain about carrying muscle weight around.

- Muscles need to be worked in order to maintain their size and vitality. If they just lay around, they'll shrink.

- It is the working (or exercising) of your muscles that burns the fat.

- The more muscle you have, the more fat you'll burn.

- Muscle is three times more dense and heavy than body fat. A pound of fat takes up three times as much space as a pound of muscle. In other words, muscle takes up only one-third the space of body fat.

- You will become more fit only by gaining more muscle, which burns more fat and calories. The only way is through proper exercise, combined with healthy, low fat eating.

Chip Off the Ol' Block

There are many reasons why shedding some pounds often feels like you're only losing ounces.

- Your genetics play a big part in predicting your body's shape and function. But that does not mean you cannot reprogram your body to shed even though your gene pool may have caused you to spread.

- The more fat you have, the longer it will take to change your body's chemistry. Be patient and keep exercising because this will eventually rev up your fat burning engine.

- Each of our bodies has a tendency to remain at some constant weight, which is known as the body's set point.

- Certain factors can raise your set point. The primary ones are lack of exercise, high fat foods, overeating, and not eating enough (starvation).

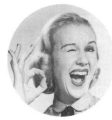

QUICK n' PAINLESS

Burn, baby, burn! Exercise keeps your body burning calories—even hours after you have finished your workout. It keeps going and going and going . . .

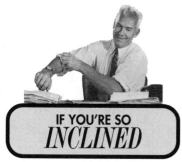

Help! I'm drowning! So, you fell in at the (heavy) end of your gene pool; it doesn't mean you're going down for the third time. You'll do swimmingly if you follow your exercise plan one stroke at a time.

- Exercise is the ultimate way to lower your body's set point.

- It is perfectly normal to experience plateaus when you are trying to lose weight. This may be a good time to change your exercise program (i.e., frequency, intensity, duration, variety). Eventually your body will continue to shed pounds.

DON'T EVEN GO THERE

There are some places you should not set foot. The first is on the road to starvation, and the second is on the bathroom scale.

Don't Bother Fasting; It Isn't Very Lasting

Ever wondered why going on a fast helped you gain weight instead of losing it?

- When you do not give your body enough energy (calories), it reacts by lowering the amount of calories it needs.

- The most efficient way to lower the body's energy requirement is by getting rid of the tissue that costs the body energy—that means your body gets rid of your muscle. When you lose muscle you lower your ability to burn fat.

- Your body also conserves its energy by storing more fat. It produces more fat-depositing enzymes to enable you to store as much fat as possible from what little fuel (calories) may be coming in.

After fasting, you are fatter than before, and it is even harder than before to lose weight.

Don't Get Weighed Down

Here's why you should not be a slave to the bathroom scale.

- Remember 1 pound of fat has 3,500 calories. Therefore, you cannot lose a pound of fat overnight. It takes time to melt away your fat stores.

- As you exercise and get fit, you will gain muscle, which is heavy and dense. Even though you may be losing fat, the scale can show a gain in weight due to your increased muscle mass. The good news is your clothes will show you've lost inches!

- Your body's water weight can fluctuate up or down, 3 to 5 pounds or more depending on how hydrated/dehydrated you are, your salt intake, or your hormone levels.

- Daily weighing will just frustrate you and can lock you into a vicious, negative cycle. Monitor your progress instead by taking tape measurements and only weighing yourself once a month.

YOUR EATING: IT'S HOW THE COOKIE CRUMBLES

Throw the food scales and calorie counters out the window. There's no time consumption or mind consumption involved. Take away the 'time' and the 'mind' and all you have left is consumption. Now that can't be too bad, can it?

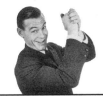

YOU'LL THANK YOURSELF LATER

Look, the sky is falling! Don't be an alarmist like Chicken Little. If your numbers on the scale aren't falling as fast as you'd like, keep in mind that muscle weighs more than fat.

Welcome to the Garden of Eatin'

If it's an apple you want, then by all means have it! Take a peek at why you won't feel so tempted.

- Almost anything goes when it comes to eating *The Lazy Way.* And pretty much everything stays too (except for unneeded fat). The key is polishing off a wide variety of wholesome, real foods. You're going to find out how easy and enjoyable eating *The Lazy Way* can be.

- Since depriving yourself is out of the question, be sure to treat yourself once a week to a delicacy that you think is soooo good but may not be so good for you. This will help keep you on your best eating behavior for the rest of the week.

- There are some foods and habits that can boost your shedding power and certain ones that can defeat it. We'll tell you more about this in Chapter 8.

- You don't have to get too drastic, but cutting back on your portions is one of the easiest ways, from an eating point of view, to attain the proper proportions.

Tracking the Fat in Just One Lap

Want a shortcut to shedding the pounds? The key is to focus on fat (pat by pat).

- It's important to know where the fat hangs out in food to avoid having it hang out somewhere on you. Here's a hint: Animal products (cheese, eggs, whole dairy, butter, meat) are loaded with it.

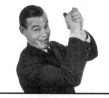

YOU'LL THANK YOURSELF LATER

You do the math! Here's an equation . . . What happens when you eat half as much and twice as slow?

- When you get rid of fat in food, you also lose taste and texture. But you can fix this without having to go to cooking school. We'll show you the brainless art of tasty low fat substitution.

- Instead of worrying about a slew of complex counting methods to lose weight, just try to have one focus—concentrate on fat. Fat really does count because it has more than double the calories of other nutrients (protein and carbohydrates).

- There are so many simple ways to cut back on fat, and we'll give them all to you in the chapters to follow.

YOUR EXERCISE: DON'T SWEAT IT!

Well, there's no getting around it—you do have to exercise. But there is exercising, and then there is exercising *The Lazy Way*. Either way will make you fit, even though the latter might take you a little longer. But what's the hurry?! As long as it's livable, right?

In Just a Heart Beat

You won't have to make your heart beat overtime to get results.

- You don't have to wear a heart monitor or count your pulse, but you do have to get to the point when you become a little heated, breathless, and sweaty.

- If you want to increase your fat burning engine, just crank up your motor and add a few spurts of higher

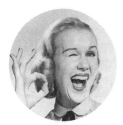

QUICK 🔘 *PAINLESS*

What color is your karma? If your cheeks are sweaty and red then your karma must be in the pink! Don't forget the mental benefits of a good physical workout . . . a clear mind, a clear conscience, and a clean bill of health.

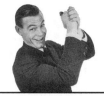

Point well taken . . . care of, that is. If you increase your exercise, avoid high fat foods, and have control over your portions, you can lower your set point. Game, set, and match!

intensity into your workout. Not the whole workout, just a few spurts.

- The more muscles you use, the less time you have to move them.

- Exercise makes your body burn more calories even hours after you have finished.

The Winning Combination

If you play the right cards in the game of exercise, you'll have a winning hand every time.

- To get fit, you need a bit of strength training (to build muscle), aerobic training (to burn fat), and stretching (to stay loose). Now, we did say just a bit.

- Thirty minutes a day is all it takes. And not even all at once. You can accumulate your exercise through-out the day, a little here, a little there.

- You don't have to give up your car or your riding mower, but if there's a way to be a tad more physi-cal in your day you should just do it. Expending a lit-tle extra energy with everything you do can add up to a bigger fat deficit.

- Your exercise program should be comfortable, con-venient, enjoyable, and effective. This way you can continue with little effort and lots of longevity.

- Exercise makes you feel great inside and out! Being active helps burn fat and calories, builds stronger muscles and bones, increases your energy and endurance, relieves stress, and reduces your risk of chronic diseases.

YOUR ATTITUDE: MINOR ADJUSTMENTS

How you feel about yourself plays an important role in how successful you are at shedding the pounds. For instance, a chip in your mouth doesn't have to become a chip on your shoulder. Changing your attitude is about letting go and lightening up. It's about how you are going to live the rest of your life . . . it sure won't be on a diet!

The State of Address

There are just a few things that will make you 'stand at attention' before you can 'stand at ease.'

- You need to know what situations trigger your taste for certain foods (i.e., popcorn at the movies, pastries at work, etc.) so that you can plan how you will deal with them. We deal with this topic in Chapter 16.

- Stress is the primary culprit for mindless eating. Luckily, the last thing you're going to be is stressed out when you shed pounds *The Lazy Way*.

- It's important to line your goals up in your sights. That way you'll hit your target every time.

You've Gotta Swap to Drop

Bad habits will only weigh you down. Are you ready to lighten your load?

- Once you are aware of your less desirable eating and exercise habits you can substitute them with

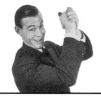

YOU'LL THANK YOURSELF LATER

Remember what mother said: "Pretty is as pretty does." The next time you go above and beyond to help someone else, remember to take pride and pleasure in the warm feeling it gives you. Health is an inside-out process.

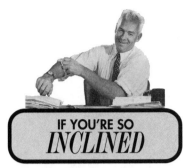

more desirable ones, whether it's what you do, what you think, or what you say.

▪ The lazy approach leaves no room for negative thoughts—they're just a waste of energy. Instead, get ready to pack the positive thoughts in. You can never have enough of those.

▪ You'll be more successful at shedding the pounds if you focus on gaining new habits rather than losing the weight.

As you can see, there's not much mystery after all to shedding some pounds *The Lazy Way*. There's no distress, difficulty, or deprivation either. Of course, you're not going to see quick results, but when it comes to weight loss, the results that come quickly never last. The lazy approach is about plugging along, making little, livable changes, shaping up effortlessly, and not letting anything get out of hand. The best thing is, you'll never have to shed those pounds again!

Getting Time on Your Side

	The Old Way	The Lazy Way
Dieting	All the time	Never again
Stressing about calories	Every single second	Not a single second
Weighing on the scale	Every day	Once a month
Exercising	At least 30 minutes a day on an organized exercise regime	30 minutes of activity every other day
Thinking about food	All the time	Only when you're hungry and need to eat

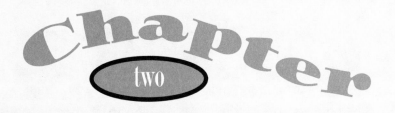

Supplies and Equipment Worth Their Weight

Don't worry, we won't burden you with running around, trying to find food scales and fancy riders or gliders. Those items are only worth the weight of the dust that should settle on them. But you will need a few particulars on hand to help you lighten your load. The great thing is you probably have most of what you need already. It's just a matter of bringing your materials all together.

Since the lazy approach to losing weight is three-pronged—eating, exercise, and attitude—you will need certain utensils for each area. First, we'll talk about the supplies that will help ease you into the process of pound shedding. Then, we'll cover what fitness equipment you'll need (most of which you probably already own). Before you know it, you'll be able to swallow it, move it, and flaunt it too!

SUPPLIES TO HELP YOU SWALLOW IT

Let's start with the stuff that will keep bad eating habits from consuming you. We'll give you supplies that will help you track, trim, measure, and spice up your foods. We promise you won't have a hard time swallowing this approach.

At Home Slim Home

In order to maintain a "Home Slim Home," you'll need supplies that cut back on fat and portions and ones that add texture and flavor. Also, you've got to have some yummy staples to prevent any snack attacks. Then there are those little inevitable inedibles—simple items you'll need to keep you on track.

Skinny Dipping for Fat

You need to have a few supplies handy that can take away some of the fat when you are preparing and/or cooking your foods. The more you can get rid of in your meals, the less you'll see on you!

These kitchen tools do wonders for degreasing your foods.

- Basters
- Ladles
- Metal racks
- Paper towels
- Slotted spoons
- Spray bottles
- Steamer

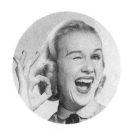

QUICK 🆕 PAINLESS

Calorie cutters unite! Gather your tools of the trade (basters, ladles, slotted spoons) into one container or handy area to be readily available for service in preparing and cooking food.

Plastic Surgery for the Proper Proportions

We all know a little plastic surgery could do wonders for our proportions, but have you ever thought about how plastic items in the kitchen could do wonders for your portions? A little plastic will keep your food contained and your appetite sustained.

Check out these plastic wares to cut into your portions.

- Baggies
- Ice cube trays
- Measuring cups
- Measuring spoons
- Small plates
- Small Tupperware containers
- Water bottles

Ammunition for Avoiding Saddlebags

You know the drill! You have to prepare to avoid a sneak food attack. Just make sure you're armed with the right provisions. You can choose your snacks depending on your taste—crunchy, salty, chewy, or sweet. Just make sure you keep then close at hand.

Here are some great snacks to avoid any hunger attacks.

- Crunchy or salty:
  - Bagel chips
  - Low fat cereals
  - Low fat crackers

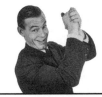

YOU'LL THANK YOURSELF LATER

Put together snack stashes at home, work, and in the car so you'll always be prepared— and you won't be tempted by the vending machine!

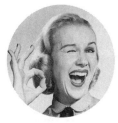

QUICK n' PAINLESS

Be a food sleuth. You don't need to buy fancy or expensive low fat or low calorie foods. Your kitchen is loaded with impostors in disguise. Substitute apples for cookies, water for soda pop, and don't forget, those pretzels aren't just for parties but do double duty as low fat chips.

- Pita chips
- Popcorn
- Pretzels
- Raw veggies
- Rice cakes
- Tortilla chips
- Chewy or sweet:
  - Applesauce
  - Bagel
  - Baked yam
  - Dried fruit
  - Energy bar
  - Fresh fruit
  - Frozen fruit juice bars
  - Licorice
  - Smoothies
  - String cheese
  - Sushi
  - Tootsie Rolls
  - Yogurt (nonfat, low fat, frozen)

Pinch an Inch for Size, Add a Dash for Taste

Zap the fat and you lose flavor and texture. Here's a bright idea: Add some tasty seasonings and substitutes to enhance your low fat cooking and baking. When you add a few condiments, you're bound to get lots of compliments.

Load up your pantry with these spices, seasonings, and substitutes (it will be hard not to load up your plate).

- Applesauce
- Broth
- Canellini beans
- Cocoa powder
- Cottage cheese (nonfat, 1% fat)
- Crushed red pepper flakes
- Egg substitute
- Egg whites
- Fresh herbs
- Fruit purées
- Garlic
- Ginger
- Horseradish
- Hot sauce
- Jalapeño
- Lemon
- Lime
- Mini chocolate chips
- Mustard (natural, grainy)
- Nonfat sour cream
- Onions
- Orange zest
- Pepper (black, cayenne, white)
- Roasted red pepper

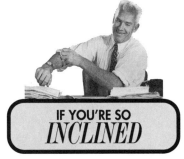

IF YOU'RE SO
INCLINED

Add a little spice to your life! Tasty seasonings and substitutions can remove the sting of less fat while adding a little zing to food! Olé!

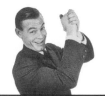

YOU'LL THANK YOURSELF LATER

Track it or you'll pack it! Planes, trains, or automobiles—where do you spend the majority of your time? Keep your food/exercise planner close at hand to track food input and energy output.

- Salsa
- Salt
- Scallions
- Seltzer water
- Shallots
- Soy sauce
- Spices
- Sun-dried tomatoes
- Vanilla extract
- Vinegars (balsamic, rice, wine)
- Worcestershire sauce
- Yogurt (nonfat, plain)

Inevitable Inedibles

There are a few supplies you should keep in your kitchen (or in the vicinity), that aren't for eating, but are necessary for tracking what you eat. These items might not be edible, but they'll sure keep you accountable.

Here's a list of mostly lists.

- Fast food list
- Fat budget
- Fat counter
- Food journal
- Grocery list
- Nutrition guides from fast food restaurants
- Treat list

SUPPLIES TO HELP YOU MOVE IT

Next, we have the exercise arena. The fitness supplies you'll need here are both basic and inexpensive. You can either use soup cans or water bottles filled with sand, buckshot, or bird seed. Or, you can get a little fancier and buy a set of dumbbells. These are available at any sporting goods store. Another alternative is elastic tubing, which you can find at a medical supply store. If you choose to work out away from home then you'll need some gear to keep you on the go.

Left to Your Own Devices

When you are left to your own devices you can find everything you need right around the house. It doesn't take much if you exercise a little creativity.

The weight these devices carry depends on how much you want to lift.

- Birdseed
- Buckshot
- Clock (or watch with second hand)
- Dumbbells (two each of 2 lbs, 5 lbs, 8 lbs, 10 lbs, 15 lbs)
- Gallon jugs
- Jump rope
- Music (stereo or portable cassette/CD player)
- Sand
- Scale

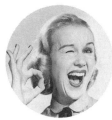

QUICK PAINLESS

Hhmmmm mmmm good idea! You need to unload the groceries anyway, so why not do a couple of reps with those soup cans before you stow them in the pantry?

- Soup cans
- Surgical tubing or rubber exercise bands (cut into 4-foot strips)
- Water bottles
- Weighted wrist bands
- Workout videos

Gear to Go

These supplies will help you stay on the move, wherever you may be. Not only will you be comfortable, you'll smell good too. So grab your gear, and you're ready to go.

Here's some gear to grip onto.

- Deodorant
- Fresh undies
- Moisture wipes
- Perfumed body spray
- Sneakers
- Sweat bands
- Towel
- Water bottle
- Workout bag
- Workout clothes (i.e., T-shirt, shorts, socks)

SUPPLIES TO HELP YOU FLAUNT IT

Are you ready for your new attitude? Then you'll need a few things to keep you focused and inspired. These supplies will help you make minor adjustments. Before you

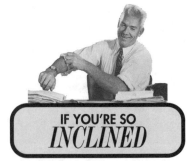

IF YOU'RE SO
INCLINED

Keep a spare set of workout gear in the trunk of your car or the corner of your closet. You never know when the spirit of adventure (and the desire to exercise) may strike. Just like the Boy Scouts, you'll want to "Be Prepared!"

know it, you'll be in a 'good' head. But, it isn't all mind over matter—you can't forget the rest of your body. Just a few accessories from the closet will leave you sleek and styling.

Matter of the Mind

These supplies may weigh a little on your mind, yet they'll leave you feeling wonderfully light at heart. Plus, surrounding yourself with mental notes, memos, and mantras will help you get your new attitude.

Here's some matter that carries a lot of weight.

- Goal sheets
- Journal
- Measurement record
- Measuring tape
- Mirror
- Motivating mantras
- Pictures
- Positive statements list
- Reward list
- Substitution list

Coming Out of the Closet

When it comes to flaunting it, there are certain supplies that every closet (or chest of drawers) should have. You want to keep a variety of these clothing elements, whether you wear them underneath or over the top.

These items will let you share it all without showing it all.

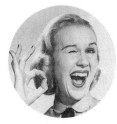

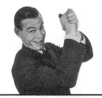

- Bathing suit wraps
- Belts
- Black basics (pants, skirts, blazers)
- Body shapers/body slimmers
- Control-top pantyhose
- Heels (low, medium, high)
- Jewelry (long necklaces)
- Long straight skirts
- Monochromatic colors
- Monochromatic ties
- Pleated pants
- Pullover sweaters
- Scarves
- Shoulder pads
- Tailored jackets (single breasted)
- Tunics/oversized shirts

YOU ONLY NEED THE KITCHEN SINK

It's a waste of time and energy to equip your home with apparatuses designed for the next Mr. or Ms. Universe. Nobody needs fancy chrome and steel fixtures to get fit, especially those of you who can do it *The Lazy Way.* After all, you would never kid yourself into thinking you'd actually get tangled up in those torture machines anyway. You know better! The fitness equipment you'll use has got to be hassle-free, nonthreatening, and efficient. So, how about the kitchen sink and a couple other pieces of furniture?!

It really can be that simple. You don't need a lot of heavy metal to challenge your muscles. Especially since you're not going to go overboard. What you do need are some basic pieces of furniture if you're going to work out in your home, along with some good resources if you choose to exercise elsewhere. For those of you who think you need more guidance and guilt (oops, we meant accountability!) with your program, we'll give you some tips on finding a personal trainer who won't brow (or butt) beat you.

It's not a bad idea to check with your doctor before starting an exercise program. Don't worry, you're not going to go overboard! But, we're going to give you some health questions to answer just in case.

"GYMMY-RIGGING" YOUR FITNESS EQUIPMENT

The beauty of working out *The Lazy Way* is that you can have a complete home gym without buying a single exercise machine. In fact, you can do most of your strength routine right at your kitchen counter. The only props you'll need are probably in your house already. One exception is a heavy block of wood, which you can pick up at your local hardware store or lumber yard.

You can find these pieces of equipment around the house.

- A bench
- A heavy block of wood
- A heavy table
- Kitchen counter

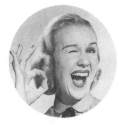

QUICK 🔘 PAINLESS

You can take this show on the road or at least out in the yard. Try doing some of your kitchen sink exercises outside using sturdy, stable pieces of patio furniture. You can better your body while watching your little darlings dig in the dirt.

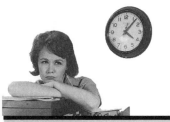

- Stairway/steps
- Two sturdy chairs

IF YOU CAN'T STAND THE HEAT, GET OUT OF THE KITCHEN

Let's say you're the type who needs to get out of the kitchen. If you want to take your fitness routine outside of your home, there are many places and organizations that offer a wide variety of activities and programs. Just make sure they are conveniently located, reasonably priced, and not too formidable. Talk to others who are already participating in the programs first to get their impressions. Try to seek out those who pride themselves on getting fit *The Lazy Way.* If most of them like it, chances are you will too.

Check out these activity resources in your community.

- Activity clubs in community (i.e., walking, hiking, biking)
- Adult education programs
- City recreation department
- Company fitness center
- Dance studios
- Health clubs
- Jazzercise
- Junior college physical education classes
- Malls (walking groups)
- Masters swimming program

A COMPLETE WASTE OF TIME

The 3 Worst Things to Do When Choosing a Health Club Are:

1. Not choose a location convenient to your home or job (if it's hard to get there you know you won't go).

2. Not check class times/gym hours to see if they will fit into your schedule.

3. Not consult with an instructor to see if they offer a class in your ability range.

- Pilatus studios
- YMCA or YWCA
- Yoga centers

IF YOU NEED YOUR HAND HELD (OR PULLED!)

For some of you, exercise would take a lot less effort if you had a trainer who came to your house to get you moving. All you'd have to do is get decent and follow instructions. There's nothing wrong with this, but realize that if you hire a personal trainer you will be investing more money as well as more time into your fitness program. You probably will not find a trainer who offers sessions less than half an hour long. The good news is when you have someone to work out with, it makes time pass more quickly.

So how do you find a fitness guru who's right for you? You should avoid any trainer who carries a whip, wears fatigues and combat boots, or is continuously flexing his or her bulging muscles. If he demands a hundred sit-ups, one-armed push-ups, and a gallon of sweat, he's not for you either. Make sure he will guide you at your level. Those who emphasize using the body instead of a bunch of equipment for resistance will be the ones most likely to give you a workout *The Lazy Way*.

You can usually find a good trainer by word of mouth (ask your friends, neighbors, and business associates), through a local health club or YMCA/YWCA, or a hospital rehabilitation center. Do make sure that you pick one who is certified by a reputable fitness organization.

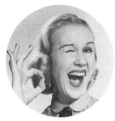

QUICK ⬤ PAINLESS

10-4 Little Buddy! Don't forget the benefits of working out with a friend, neighbor, or co-worker. Just 10 minutes a day four times a week can have you roaring down the road to success in no time.

Here's a list of the best known ones:

- Aerobics and Fitness Association of America (AFAA)
- American College of Sports Medicine (ACSM)
- American Council on Exercise (ACE)
- The Cooper Clinic
- National Academy of Sports Medicine (NASM)
- National Strength and Conditioning Association (NSCA)

ARE YOU READY TO GET SET AND GO, OR DO YOU HAVE A STUBBED TOE?

Exercising *The Lazy Way* should not pose any problem or hazard. But it is always a good idea to get a check-up before you embark on an exercise program (no matter how lazy it is). It's also important to discuss any restriction your doctor may have for you.

In order to help you get a general idea as to whether you are ready to exercise, we've given you a little health quiz to take. (Don't worry, it's open book!)

Just answer yes or no to the following list of questions:

1. Has your doctor ever said you have heart trouble?

2. Has your doctor ever said your blood pressure was too high?

3. Does walking up a flight of stairs make you short of breath?

4. Do you often feel faint or have spells of dizziness?

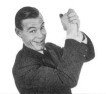

YOU'LL THANK YOURSELF LATER

Take a moment to make an appointment with your doctor and get a check-up before you begin your exercise program. It helps to have a green light before you go.

5. Do you ever have pain, pressure, or tightness in your chest brought on by exertion?

6. Has your doctor ever told you that you have a bone, joint, muscular, or vein problem (i.e., arthritis, gout, bad back, or varicose veins) that is aggravated or made worse by exercising?

7. Are you over 65 and not accustomed to moderate exercise?

8. Do you smoke more than a pack of cigarettes a day?

9. Are you more the 50 pounds overweight?

10. Is there a good physical reason, not mentioned above, why you should not start an exercise program?

   If you answered 'yes' to one or more questions, consult your doctor before increasing your physical activity. If you answered 'no' to all of the questions, then you can be reasonably sure that you are physically ready to exercise *The Lazy Way*. Of course, you'll begin slowly and increase your activity gradually (just be careful not to stub your toe!).

   Whether you work out with a personal trainer, at a club, or amongst your own furniture, be sure to keep it simple. Using your body with just a few props is not only basic, it's convenient. It is actually one of the most effective ways to strengthen your muscles and improve your coordination and balance. So remember, nothing fancy! Just do what works for you and what will keep you working out.

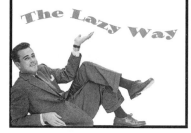

Congratulations! You've given yourself a health quiz! Now give yourself a break and enjoy a nice walk in the park!

The Lazy Way

Getting Time on Your Side

	The Old Way	The Lazy Way
Skimming off the grease	5 minutes	30 seconds
Getting yourself some dumbbells	Up to several hours	No more than a few minutes
Gathering your workout gear	5 to 8 minutes	30 seconds
Strength training	At the gym	At home
	Getting there: 10 minutes	Getting there: 0 minutes
	Session time: 30 minutes	Session time: 15 minutes
Personal training	Their place	Your place
	Getting there: 10 minutes	Getting there: 0 minutes
	Session time: 30 minutes	Session time: 30 minutes
Cardiovascular training	Aerobics class	Around the block
	Getting there: 10 minutes	Getting there: 0 minutes
	Session time: 60 minutes	Session time: 30 minutes

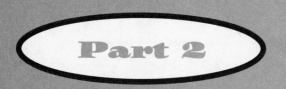

Part 2

Take a Bite Out of Time

Are You Too Lazy to Read Take a Bite Out of Time?

1 You think that trimming down means starving yourself for a week. ☐ yes ☐ no

2 You think that watching what you eat means you have to spend hours in the grocery aisle comparing nutritional values on the back of every box. ☐ yes ☐ no

3 Cooking healthy always seems as if it would take too long and definitely seems too complicated to even try. ☐ yes ☐ no

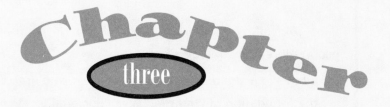

Do It or Diet

You probably think shedding pounds *The Lazy Way* means following an eating plan that's already laid out for you. Like the ol' dry routine, for instance—dry toast, dry salads, and dry chicken! Well, following someone else's meal concoctions is the furthest away you can get from effortless eating. Rather, you want to embrace your own food habits and quirks. They've been with you much too long for you to abandon them now. Just sink your teeth into the following simple "to do" tips, and you'll avoid the struggle of a diet.

The pointers that we give you in this chapter encompass more than just your eating. After all, your exercise and attitude also play an important role in your success at losing weight. Take your time and see how you can incorporate these do-ahead tips, so that you can prepare yourself for effortless and permanent shedding.

GIVE YOURSELF YOUR DAILY BREAD AND BUTTER

Your best nourishment comes from real, wholesome foods, and the easiest way to track how much you should eat is to

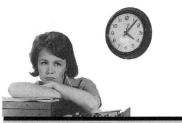

allot yourself a number of servings from each food group. Here's how it works . . .

■ Intend to make breads, cereals, legumes, and grains the foundation of your diet. Give yourself 6 to 11 servings* per day. Always select at least half of your grains and starches from whole-grain sources.

* Note: Don't sweat serving sizes too much right now. As you continue through the book, we'll be showing you lazy ways to size up your portions. But don't worry! There won't be any weighing or calorie counting charts involved!

■ Figure on having only a few fruits a day. Even though they are a great source of fiber, vitamins, and phytochemicals, they are high in natural sugar, and so they should be eaten in moderation. Give yourself two to four servings per day.

■ Plan to get in plenty of veggies. The darker or more colorful a vegetable is, the more nutritious it is for you. Whether you eat them raw or cooked, give yourself four to six servings per day.

■ Don't forget the dairy group. Dairy products are rich in protein and calcium but can also be high in fat. So stick to the nonfat choices. If you're allergic to milk or dairy foods, soy-based products are a good substitute. Give yourself two servings per day.

■ Reckon on using meats, eggs, cheeses, and nuts in moderation. Start thinking of meat and other high fat protein foods as condiments rather than the main attraction of your meals. Give yourself two servings (4 to 6 ounces) per day.

- Don't estimate on the extras. You need to limit the amount of fat and sugar you add to your food because they have lots of calories and little else. Give yourself two to three servings of fat and no more than 8 to 15 servings of added sugar per day.

- Aim to avoid alcohol. Alcoholic drinks (1 ounce hard liquor, 4 ounces wine, 12 ounces beer) are highly caloric, and these calories offer no nutrients. Even though alcohol doesn't contain fat, it does interfere with your body's ability to burn fat. So try to limit yourself to no more than four drinks a week.

- Work on getting in lots of water. This wonder tonic is 100% natural and totally calorie free. Stock your fridge, car, and workout bag with water bottles (filled, of course), and make it a habit to carry a water bottle around with you. Give yourself at least eight servings per day, and more if you're in the heat.

- Contemplate taking a multivitamin-mineral supplement as added insurance for good health. (Remember, nothing beats real food for providing you with the nutrients you need.) Choose a supplement that has no artificial colors or fillers and has no more than 100 to 150% of the recommended daily allowance (RDA) for every essential nutrient.

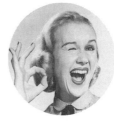

QUICK ⫿⫿ PAINLESS

Cut that out! Carry a food guide with you that indicates the grams of fat in your favorite fast food meals. You'll be able to cut into your waistline without cutting into your wait time.

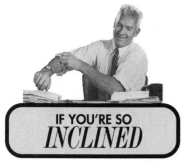

Happy trails to you! Blaze your own trail by mixing your own special blend of low fat selections to make an on-the-go snack. Try combinations of tried and true favorites: pretzels, popcorn, toasted cereal, or stake a claim to your own winning combination.

JACK SPRAT COULD EAT NO FAT, BUT DON'T YOU SETTLE FOR THAT

We want you to cut back on fat, but not give it up completely! Follow these fat-trimming tips for some quick ways to eat lean. (We promise you'll still want to lick the platter clean!)

- Buy a pump spray bottle and fill it with olive or canola oil. Keep this handy for sautéeing, roasting, stir-frying, and/or grilling.

- Always trim all visible fat off of meats before cooking.

- Leave the skin on poultry for cooking. This will keep the meat moist and will not add any extra fat to it. Do make sure you take it off before eating though. Then, it would be finger lickin' good for you.

- Here's a tip you can dip into right away. Always ask for dressings and sauces in a separate dish on the side. That way, you can dip your fork in them to get a touch of flavor with each bite. You'll be surprised how much goo will be left behind.

- Skim the fat off the surface of soups, stocks/broths, stews, or sauces before you serve them. You can use a ladle or baster, but the easiest thing to do is put the pot in the refrigerator for a while. As the fat cools, it will harden, and then you can scoop it right off the top.

- Put yourself on a fat budget. Ladies, try to stay between 27 to 44 grams of fat. And you guys need around 44 to 62 fat grams. Spread these throughout the day. Limit your saturated fat intake to $1/3$ of your daily fat grams (9 to 20 grams). You can buy a basic fat counter at the book store to help you figure out where the fat hangs out in foods.

SHOP SO YOU'LL DROP

Buyers beware! Going into grocery stores can be hazardous to your health and your hips. But, not if you follow these simple shopping tips.

- Before you step foot in the grocery store, give yourself some ground rules—never shop when you are hungry, in a hurry, or under the influence of hormones!

- Shop "around" for the healthiest foods. In most stores, the real, wholesome foods can be found on the perimeter. So stick around the outside aisles of the store, and you can avoid the sea of packaged and processed products in the middle aisles.

- If you have to venture into those middle aisles, be sure to read food labels. The main items to look at are the serving size, the calories, and the fat grams (total and saturated). Check out the ingredients too—they are always listed by weight, starting with most and ending with the least.

- Be suspicious of sugar-loading in your boxed food products, especially breakfast foods and snack bars. Watch for words ending in "-ose" (dextrose, sucrose,

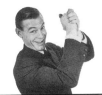

YOU'LL THANK YOURSELF LATER

Just say no! If you don't need it, don't get it. Type up a basic grocery list, make copies, highlight what you need each week, and don't deviate. You'll come home lighter of mind but not of pocket.

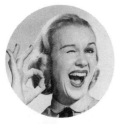

etc.) and sweet ingredients like corn syrup, corn syrup solids, cane juice, honey, and brown sugar.

■ Scope out the health food or natural/whole food stores in your neighborhood. They will have an abundance of wholesome choices for breakfast, lunch, dinner, and don't forget dessert.

■ Check to see if you have a farmer's market in your area. This is where you'll find the best selection of fruits and vegetables. After fresh produce, frozen ones are your next best choice, then choose the canned variety (low sodium/no syrup).

THERE'S NO NEED TO SNEAK AROUND FOR SNACKS

Snacking is an essential part of *The Lazy Way* to shed some pounds. So don't feel guilty about grabbing a snack, especially when you incorporate these snacking guidelines.

■ Preplan your snack times so that you snack smart and avoid overeating at meal times.

■ Organize one cupboard for your snacks. Keep the healthier choices on the bottom where they're easier to reach and the not-so-healthy ones up high.

■ Always keep fresh fruit out in a bowl or a basket.

■ Have a drawer in your refrigerator stocked with cleaned and cut veggies like carrots, celery, broccoli, and bell peppers. Put a nonfat dip in the drawer to keep them company.

- Don't forget to fill your freezer with a supply of fruit juice bars for something cold and sweet. Nonfat frozen yogurt hits the spot too.

- Keep a couple of healthy snacks in your car and at the office.

LIST OR BE LISTLESS

You'd probably be lost without a list of 'to dos.' That's why we're giving you these ideas for making some helpful lists that won't leave you listless.

- Create your own personal grocery list of everything you buy from the store. Then make copies of it so you can use a clean list every time you shop. That way, you only have to check off what you need each time.

- Make up a list of all your favorite fast food spots and then choose the items at each place that are low in fat (consult the nutrition guides provided by each fast food restaurant). Make some extra copies so that you can keep this list in your car and your purse. Promise yourself that you will order items only from this list.

- We probably all have some high fat, sugary treats we just can't live without. The key is to make sure they don't stick around (on us) too long. Take a look at the chart at the end of Chapter 12, which shows the amount of minutes it takes to burn off different goodies. Choose your favorites and their activity equivalents from this chart to make your own

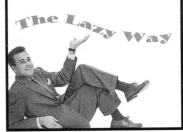

Congratulations! Without breaking a sweat you have just organized yourself and your supplies one cupboard closer to a healthier, slimmer you. Enjoy your new found freedom of choice by selecting and savoring whichever low fat snack you crave!

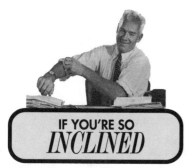

What's for dinner? Design five basic menus, write down all the ingredients needed on the back of each sheet, make copies, and keep them convenient in your briefcase, purse, or car. Next stop, stressless shopping. It's the next best thing to a drive-thru grocery store.

personal list of treats. This will remind you that if you choose it, you've gotta use it.

- Make up a list of 10 nonfood-related rewards that make you feel special, and turn to this list when you feel you deserve a treat!

A FEW EXERCISE "TO DOS" BEFORE YOU JUST DO IT

Don't worry! We're not going to ask you to work hard before you even work out. Rather, we think the following "to dos" will ease you into your exercise.

- If you choose to make your own dumbbells, you will need to get four small water bottles (16-ounce) and two large jugs with handles (gallon milk jugs). Fill them with water, sand, birdseed, or buck shot (fillers are in order of increasing weight). Weigh the bottles on a scale to create two 3-pound weights, two 5-pound weights, and two 10-pound weights.

- Designate a small area for your exercise and keep your fitness supplies there. If you have hard wood or cement floors you'll want to get a little rug to make it more comfortable.

- Keep a set of workout clothes, fresh undies, and sneakers in a workout bag along with an extra set of your toiletries. Put this bag by the door or in the trunk of your car so you won't forget it that easily.

- Buy an extra pair of sneakers and keep them at work just in case you have a chance to take an active break.

- Check the Yellow Pages to see what clubs or fitness organizations are in your area. Give them a call to see what activities they offer.

- Join forces with some of your buddies to boost camaraderie and help keep you honest.

- Schedule your chunks of exercise time into your planner every day. Whether it's 10 minutes or 3, you need to put it in writing so that you will keep that appointment with yourself.

CRUISE THROUGH YOUR CHRONICLES

It's important to keep track of things like portions, inches, and feelings. Here are some simple ways to do just that.

- Go out and buy yourself a journal. This book will end up being just as important as your "little black" one.

- Keep a food journal for a few days, including a day on the weekend. Write down what you eat and include the amounts, the time, and how you feel as you're eating. This will give you an idea of your eating patterns and challenges.

- Take your measurements. Check your chest, waist, hip, and thigh, and record the numbers in your journal. You can recheck these every four to six weeks (that's a good time to weigh yourself too). If you are able, try to have your body fat tested every few months. Record your progress in your journal.

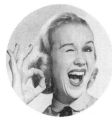

QUICK ⟨n⟩ PAINLESS

Don't be a dumbbell, make one! Milk jugs with handles, bottles of water . . . find 'em, fill 'em, and flex 'em.

Getting Time on Your Side

	The Old Way	The Lazy Way
Skinning your poultry	5 minutes	A big, fat egg (0 minutes)
Planning your grocery list	5 minutes	1 minute
Searching for a snack at work	5 minutes	30 seconds
Skimming the fat off your soup	15 minutes and a big mess	10 minutes and no mess
Ordering at a fast food restaurant	15 minutes	5 minutes
Planning dinner	20 minutes	2 seconds

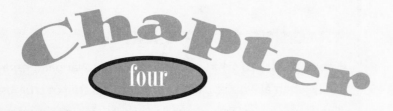

Chapter four

Gotta Minute?

We live in a hurried world, where time speeds by in a blur, and the only chance we have to get anything done is during the commercials. Then it seems we run around like a chicken looking for its head. Are we doomed to always be in this state of frenzy? Now, don't get your feathers too ruffled. It doesn't have to be that way. We'll show you some shortcuts that will just take a minute. We promise you won't need a second more.

The problem with our fast-paced society is that there is too much pressure pulling us apart and not enough time to keep ourselves together. That's why it's imperative that you stay on the lazy path. It will lead to tracking in a twinkling and plenty of moments to unwind. You'll save time with planned leftovers and stay focused with just a few jots in your journal.

These shortcuts will save you lots of time and energy. You'll be able to put it to good use when you discover a dozen easy ways to make the most of your muscles. So, what do you think? Gotta minute?

Before you swallow it, follow it . . . how far down the processed family tree is your food choice? One step away from mother nature is best (uncooked fruits and vegetables, whole grains). Anything that's a second or third cousin to fresh may as well be forgotten (and cut out of your will . . . power).

TRACKING IN A TWINKLING

Keeping track of what you eat can be a royal pain, especially when all you're used to noticing is a trail of crumbs. That's why we recommended that you concentrate mostly on sizing up your servings (see Chapter 7). This will keep your tracking to a minimum. But, there are a few you'll want to keep tabs on. We'll show you efficient ways to track items like water, fat grams, sugar, and grocery needs.

Stick to this track and you'll avoid a stress attack.

- Find a designated spot for your grocery list so that family members can check off any items you are out of or need.

- Quickly scan the ingredients of food labels. If you find that you can't pronounce most of the words, then you probably are looking at a food that isn't too wholesome.

- If you want to track your sugar intake from a nutrition label, look at the line that reads "Sugars" under "Total Carbohydrate." Take the number of grams of sugar and divide it by four. (There are 4 grams of sugar in 1 teaspoon.) This will give you the number of teaspoons of sugar in one serving.

- You can keep track of your water intake by filling a 64-ounce pitcher up and putting it in the fridge. You'll know you haven't drunk all of your water until it's empty.

- When choosing a boxed snack, try to stay within 100 calories and 1 to 2 grams of fat. Keep prepared or frozen meals around 500 to 600 calories and 10 fat grams.

- On a small piece of paper, divvy up your fat grams between your meals and snacks (remember to keep your budget around 27 to 44/44 to 62 grams). Plan to get most of your fat grams during the first part of the day. Now take this paper and place it somewhere where you can't miss it.

SAVE SOME TIME WITH PLANNED LEFTOVERS

Another day goes by and the question pops up once again . . . "What's for dinner?" It's a question that can cause daily stress, sometimes to the point of making you not want to go home and face it. Yet, somehow you manage to throw together a meal most of the time.

If you plan your meals (especially the big one) before hand, you can make healthy choices and save a lot of time. Better yet, if you plan your meals from leftovers, you can save even more time. The key is to make extra when you are cooking certain basics and then use them in various ways for different meals.

These tips show you how to squeeze more out of your foods so you won't be squeezed for time.

- Cook extra pasta. Rub your hands with a little olive oil and toss the planned over portion to keep it from sticking. Keep refrigerated, then use in salads or soups.

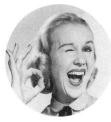

QUICK ⬛ PAINLESS

Reincarnation isn't only for Shirley MacLaine. Your veggies and side dishes can have an encore performance and come back to life (and the dinner table) tomorrow night as well. Monday's steamed broccoli can become part of Tuesday's pasta primavera. Be creative with your cooking!

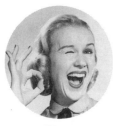

- Bake extra potatoes. They'll cook on their own while you're having dinner, and they keep well in the fridge. Use the extras in soups and side dishes.

- Roast red bell peppers, then peel them and remove the seeds and veins; purée them, plain or with a little olive oil and garlic; freeze in ice cube trays then pack the cubes into air tight freezer bags. Use for flavor boosters in soups and sauces.

- Make a quick, zippy sauce of tomatoes, onion, garlic, and a touch of olive oil. To half, add red pepper flakes, cilantro, and lime; place over broiled chicken and tuck into warm corn tortillas. The next day, mix the reserved half with fresh basil or herbs and a little parmesan and toss with pasta; or, place on top of Boboli with fresh veggies and broil it for a quick pizza.

- Purchase a roasted chicken from the deli section of your grocery store. Cut yourself (and your family) a piece for the first night then shred the leftover chicken meat for tacos, soups, sandwiches, or casseroles.

TAKE A MOMENT TO UNWIND

Remember, stress is one of the primary causes for mindless eating. Therefore, you need to do what you can to diminish your stress, or at least control it. Now, it just doesn't make sense to stress out about how you're going to get rid of your stress, so relax, take a deep breath, and follow a few tips from us.

These simple ways to unwind won't leave you spinning.

- Whether you just came home from a long day at work or finished putting away the dinner dishes, give yourself a little time to unwind by walking around the block once or twice.

- Take an ice cube and rub it on the back of your neck and your temples. This will melt away your tension in no time.

- When we sit for a long time, we tend to hunch over into question marks. Take a moment to straighten yourself back into an exclamation point. Stand up and pretend you are being pulled from a string on top of your head. Feel your spine lengthening as you press your chin up and shoulders down.

- It's important to take some quiet time for yourself. Here's a meditation exercise that will just take a minute. Sit up straight with your legs and arms uncrossed. Close your eyes and breathe deeply. Now begin visualizing the colors of the rainbow, starting at your feet. Imagine the colors changing as they go up through your body to your head.

- Go visit nature. She is the queen of playgrounds. Try to get to a beach, mountain, forest, meadow, or river at least once a month.

- Laugh whenever you can! Laughter stirs up your insides and lightens your mood. It's one of the best ways to dissipate stress.

Congratulations! You've mastered the art of unwinding in a way that is good for you! Buy yourself some flowers so you can stop and smell the roses!

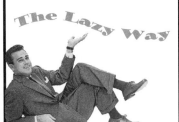

The Lazy Way

JUST A JOT IN THE DARK

Keeping a journal is like having a special friend by your side. It allows you to look inside yourself and express how you feel without constraint. Sometimes it may take a while to put your thoughts and goals on paper, but for the most part, your journal keeping can be kept to just a jot in the dark (although daylight would probably be better).

The hardest part about keeping a journal is making it a habit, and this can take a lot of time. That's why we're going to give you some guidelines to help speed up the process.

Follow these tips, and you'll shorten your journey toward completing your journal.

▪ Find a special spot for your journal and always keep it there when you aren't using it. Also, choose a quiet place where you can write. That way you won't waste any time getting down to business.

▪ Pick a specific time to write in your journal. Whether it's first thing in the morning or the last thing you do at night, having a time carved out just for journal writing will make this task less of a hassle and more of a routine.

▪ Boost your morale by taking a moment to read an inspirational quote or story every day. Jot down any meaningful quotes or sayings in your journal.

▪ You will be making promises to yourself in your journal (see Chapters 14 through 16), and it's important to reinforce them daily. Just cut to the 'paste'

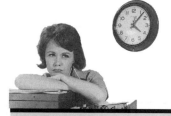

A COMPLETE WASTE OF TIME

The 3 Worst Things NOT to Do When Writing in Your Journal:

1. Find a quiet moment.

2. Take time to do it.

3. Look for a peaceful spot.

and repeat your promises in the mirror after each time you brush your teeth.

- Take a minute to schedule your measurement dates in your planner. Space them out every four to six weeks. That way, time won't slip by without you measuring your progress.

A DOZEN WAYS TO MAKE THE MOST OF YOUR MUSCLES IN A MINUTE

Gotta minute? Then you have time to sneak some calorie-burning activities into your routine. Making the most of your muscles whenever you have a spare moment will definitely make a dent in your pound shedding. All it takes is a little creativity.

Here are some easy, painless moves for your muscles that will just take a minute.

- Skip to your mailbox.
- Do a wall-sit.
- Perform the sun salutation (yoga).
- Lie down, hug your knees to your chest, and rock gently side to side.
- Do the "hokey-pokey."
- Park farther away from your destination.
- Beat cake batter with a wooden spoon.
- Take the stairs.
- Do jumping jacks or jump rope.
- Knead your dough a minute longer.

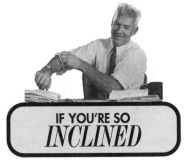

IF YOU'RE SO INCLINED

New and improved. Try doing your daily chores at a slightly quicker pace than usual to rev up your calorie burners. Trot the dog, sprint to the mailbox, and dance down the driveway. You'll use up just a little breath and a lot more calories.

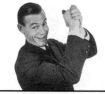

- Grab some friends and do the can-can.
- Do walking lunges to get your paper.

These are just some ideas to get you started. We're sure you can come up with dozens of your own.

Getting Time on Your Side

	The Old Way	**The Lazy Way**
Reading a food label	2 minutes	30 seconds
Salvaging leftovers	3 minutes	30 seconds
Writing in your journal	10 to 20 minutes	5 to 8 minutes
Planning dinner	1 hour every day	30 minutes once a week
Buying groceries	20 minutes, twice a day every week	30 minutes once a week
Beating stress	Impossible!	A few minutes, in a quiet spot

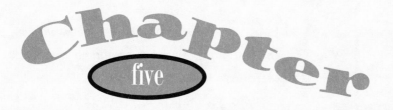

Chapter five

The Two-Second Tidy

Hold on! It will just take two seconds . . . Yes, it's probably not the most exciting thing to have to tidy up, but it doesn't have to be tedious. Remember to stick to the lazy approach—a little lick here and a smooth swipe there—and you'll have everything cleaned up in no time.

The two-second tidy doesn't just mean you'll be degreasing your food and forehead. Tidying up loose food ends will keep you from becoming a pack rat. Following up on measurements and goals helps keep you clear and uncluttered. Last but not least, tidying up the house is just one more way to burn extra calories.

LICKETY-SPLIT! YOU'VE GOT FAT LICKED

Fat is a sticky character. It not only adheres to food but loves to latch on to our bodies too. Luckily, there are ways to peel fat away from foods before we eat them. (If only we could peel it off our bodies that easily!)

This is where your kitchen tools (see Chapter 2, "Supplies and Equipment Worth Their Weight"), come in handy. They'll

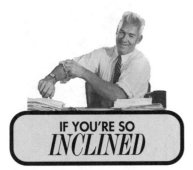

Plan ahead! Leftovers from tonight's dinner could make an easy casserole on Saturday—two meals for the price of one!

help you blot, skim, and extract the grease with ease. You'll be able to tidy up without having to worry about fat sticking around.

Here's how to get fat licked, lickety-split:

- When you roast or broil meat in the oven, first line a pan with foil, then place a metal rack on top. Stick the meat on the rack and the fat will drip onto the foil. When you're through cooking, you can just roll up the foil and throw it away.

- It's much easier and cleaner to leave the skin on poultry, taking it off after it's cooked rather than when it's raw.

- If you want to get rid of the fat and skin of uncooked poultry, use two baggies as gloves. This will keep your hands from getting slimy.

- Always blot off the oil with a paper towel when you are preparing bacon or other greasy foods.

- Keep your canned broths in the refrigerator. This will harden the fat so you can easily glean it from the top when you're ready to use it.

IT JUST TAKES A SEC TO SAVE YOURSELF FROM SECONDS

It's usually not the minutes we spend eating that makes it hard to shed the pounds, but rather the seconds (we may take) during that time. So, it's important to spend a second or two figuring out how to deal with any abundance of food that may surround you. Whether it's your kid's leftover sandwich or the chips and salsa at dinner, you need to come up with a game plan to prevent you from over indulging.

Here are some tips to tick off the seconds.

- There's no commandment that says, "Thou shalt eat thy offspring's unscathed victuals." So, don't give your kids' leftovers a second thought. Throw them in the fridge, the garbage, or the dog's bowl.

- Ever notice that tasting while cooking dinner can add up to a meal? Keep a bowl of hot soapy water handy to dip your utensils in immediately after you stir the pot, so you won't go overboard on the savoring.

- You can save yourself from getting stuffed on chips or bread at a restaurant. The key is to have one handful or slice and then ask the waitress to take it away.

- Decide to tidy up only half your entrée when eating out. Immediately divide your dish and send the remainder with the waiter for a doggy bag. Then you'll be able to enjoy your meal twice as much.

- Decadent desserts can be deadly, but you can stay in control if you take a couple bites and then dirty the rest with some salt and pepper.

THREE SWIPES AND THE SWEAT IS OUTTA HERE

It's no fun being sweaty, so the sooner you can swipe it off the better, right? Fortunately, you'll be working out *The*

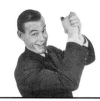

YOU'LL THANK YOURSELF LATER

Here's a tip. Don't be intimidated into eating more than you should by fancy surroundings or a haughty headwaiter. He'll be impressed by your self-control.

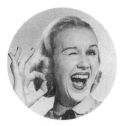

Lazy Way, so you won't have as much sweat to contend with. But, we'll show you how to remove even the slightest drop of perspiration.

These tip-offs will keep you in the sweat-free zone.

- When you are on the teeny plan (10 three-minute chunks of exercise time), the most you'll need for tidying up is a moisture wipe. You should try to keep moisture wipes in a variety of places—workout bag, glove box, purse, and desk drawers.

- If you choose to do the tiny plan (six five-minute chunks), you can clean up easily with a wet towel. Just wet half of it to swipe your sweat, then dry yourself off with the other half.

- The little plan (three 10-minute chunks) will get you sweaty and may be a little smelly too. If you don't have time for a quick shower, spruce yourself up with a wet towel and then add a touch of deodorant and/or body spray.

- If you don't want to feel the sweat drip from your body, position yourself in front of a fan. This will keep you dry and it will feel like you are tidying up as you are working out.

- Wear a terrycloth headband and/or wristbands when you work out, especially when it's hot. These will definitely help sop up the sweat.

FULL TILT FOLLOW-UPS

Follow-ups are important for keeping in touch with your pound shedding progress. It's so easy to shift into automatic mode and forget about things like looking toward goals and practicing new habits. That's why you need to "put it into park" and take some time to reflect on your performance.

These full tilt follow-ups will keep you from crashing.

■ Set aside a few minutes at the end of every day to reflect on how you are staying on track and/or what might have led you astray. Enter your reflections in your journal—this will keep you close to your progress.

■ When you shed pounds *The Lazy Way*, you are continually setting and achieving little goals. Chart your daily, weekly, and monthly goals in your planner; and when they become accomplishments, jot them down in your journal.

■ Follow up on your pound shedding progress every four to six weeks with your tape measure. Taking these measurements (along with a body composition analysis) is the best way to monitor your shrinkage.

TIDY UP TO TRIM DOWN

We want you to look at your household chores in a different light. Don't think of them as a bothersome nuisance but rather an efficient way to burn more calories. Doing household tasks as a form of exercise will help you get your work done better and faster too. And you wondered why Cinderella never complained about her chores!

Dance your way through your daily duties and work out too! Add a little disco to your dusting, some bop to your mop, and waltz through your wash.

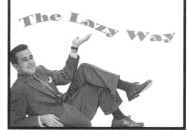

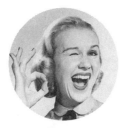

QUICK n' PAINLESS

It's easy to be efficient if you can kill two birds with one stone! Combine your daily tasks with some exercises, and you'll get organized and fit at the same time!

Here are some ways to turn the work around the house into a workout.

- Turn the stereo on the next time you clean the house. Choose music that is so snappy it makes you zip right through your chores.

- Do calf raises the next time you wash dishes or iron the clothes.

- Incorporate lunges into your vacuuming routine.

- Flip the cushions on your couch and chairs once a week. If you're really ambitious, go ahead and flip your mattress weekly too.

- Don't stack dishes when you clear the table. Remove them one at a time.

- Actually wash the dishes before you put them in the dishwasher.

- Each time you have to go up your stairs, run back down and do them again.

- Pull a dozen weeds from your yard every day.

- Say good-bye to your dryer and start hanging your clothes on a line to dry.

Getting Time on Your Side

	The Old Way	The Lazy Way
Clean up after your workout	20 to 30 minutes	3 to 8 minutes
Skimming fat off broth	2 minutes	10 seconds
Preparing your entrée	15 to 20 minutes	8 to 10 minutes
Keeping cool while you work out	Impossible!	No sweat!
Getting rid of grease	3 hours scraping the pans	2 minutes after cooking (we love aluminum foil!)
Draining fat off greasy foods	20 minutes	2 minutes

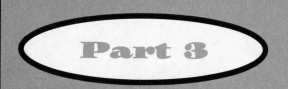

Part 3

Now You're Sizzlean'!

Are You Too Lazy to Read Now You're Sizzlean'?

1 You feel as if you spend more time feeling bad about yourself than you do feeling good. ☐ yes ☐ no

2 "Health food" directly translates to "rabbit food." ☐ yes ☐ no

3 This sounds familiar: "I'm too tired to start today, I'll start exercising tomorrow." ☐ yes ☐ no

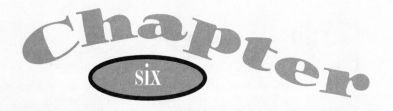

Not as Creamy but Just as Dreamy

Let's face it! Fat makes foods taste good. Not just good, but downright delicious! And then, there's the heavenly texture—crispy, flaky, silky, or smooth. It's hard to imagine that foods with less fat can still be scrumptious, but it can be done. We'll show you how to make your entrées and desserts not as creamy but just as dreamy.

This won't take much effort on your part . . . only a little awareness and some great substitutions. Remember, the whole reason why we're even suggesting this is because fat has more than double the calories of any other food. Fat also is stored more readily; therefore, cutting back the fat in your recipes is a sure way to make a dent in the fat on your body.

So, get ready to discover where the fat hangs out in foods and how to easily master the art of low fat substitution. Then, you can sit back and enjoy your meals without missing an ounce of the fat.

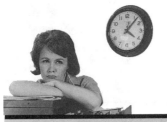

The 3 Worst Times to Try Substituting Low Fat or Nonfat Ingredients in Your Recipes:

1. When you are baking (and the amount of ingredients called for has to be exact).

2. When you would lose the essence of the dish (eat a smaller portion instead).

3. When it needs to be perfect (try it out on family before you present it to friends).

LET IT ALL HANG OUT

Fat can be pretty sneaky when it comes to hiding out in our snacks and meals. Of course, sometimes it doesn't care—leaving a trail of grease spots wherever it goes. But other times it fools us—sinking into foods without a trace.

You don't need to buy a magnifying glass or hire a detective. We'll show you where fat hangs out in different foods within the following lists. Whether it's a little or a lot, knowing fat's favorite hide-outs will keep this greasy character from getting the 'butter' of you.

The Not So Fatty Fare

These goods are low on fat's list of hang-outs. They contain about 3 to 5 grams of fat per average serving.

- Avocado
- Buttermilk
- Chicken breast (no skin)
- Clams
- Low fat cheese
- Low fat cottage cheese
- Low fat crackers
- Low fat potato chips
- Low fat tortilla chips
- Low fat yogurt
- Parmesan cheese
- Sherbet

- Turkey (white meat)
- Waffles/pancakes (no butter)

The Fattier Fare

You'll find a bit more of the squishy stuff hidden in these foods. They each have around 5 to 10 grams of fat per average serving. Be shrewd and consume this fare in moderation.

- All oils (1 teaspoon)
- Beef
- Breaded/fried fish
- Butter
- Cheese (regular)
- Chicken (w/skin or fried)
- Chips (regular)
- Cookies
- Corn nuts
- Crackers (regular)
- Cream cheese
- Crisco
- Dark turkey meat
- Eggs
- Feta cheese
- French toast (no butter)
- Granola
- Lamb

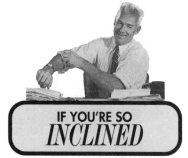

IF YOU'RE SO INCLINED

Solid gold. If you have some "oldies but goodies" that are high fat family favorites, don't throw out the dish with the dishwater . . . lighten them up! Take a few moments to modify your recipes with low fat substitutes for those high fat ingredients. You'll retain the great taste instead of the extra weight.

- Lard
- Lobster
- Low fat milk
- Macaroni and cheese
- Margarine
- Mayonnaise
- Miracle whip
- Most frozen dinners
- Olives
- Peanut butter
- Popcorn (oil popped)
- Pork
- Prepackaged pasta/rice dinners
- Pudding
- Salad dressings (most)
- Salmon
- Sausage
- Tahini

The Fattiest Fare

Fat hardly disguises itself in these foods. They are loaded with more than 10 grams of fat per average serving. Choose these foods sparingly.

- All nuts
- Bologna
- Cakes

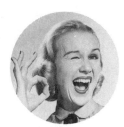

QUICK n° PAINLESS

Presentation is every-thing. Just because your food lost fat and calories, doesn't mean it lost its sense of style. How you present it is as important as what's in it. A pretty plate will please your palate.

- Candy bars
- Chili
- Chocolate
- Croissants
- Doughnuts
- French fries
- Hash browns
- Hot dogs
- Ice cream
- Most fast foods
- Most sauces
- Pesto
- Pizza
- Quiche
- Sunflower seeds
- Trail mixes

THE BUTCHER, THE BAKER, AND THE LOW FAT MAKER

We did promise that you don't need to go to cooking school to learn how to lower the fat in your recipes. You won't have to spend hours slaving in your kitchen either. Here are some simple techniques that will help you adapt your favorite dishes and desserts into low fat, high-flavor creations.

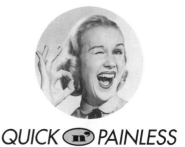

QUICK ʘ PAINLESS

Just a teaspoon of oil makes the fat content go down. Remember to spray it, not pour it!

Cutting the Fat Without Butchering Your Meals

You probably have never questioned the amount of fat (butter, oil, etc.) a recipe calls for. After all, it's the fat that makes it taste so delicious, right? Well, the good news is a little fat goes a long way. Here are a bunch of ways to ease up on the grease without destroying your recipes.

- Give up the free pouring of oil and start spraying it on. Use your spray bottle for sautéeing, browning, grilling, or roasting.

- Instead of eating fried tortilla, potato, pita, or bagel chips, make your own using your sprayer. Just place your favorite on a cookie sheet; spray and season on both sides; and bake at 400 degrees, turning occasionally, until golden brown and crispy.

- Most entrée recipes call for more oil than is needed. You can lower this amount by figuring on 1 teaspoon for each person the dish will serve. For example, if you are feeding six people and the recipe calls for $1/4$ cup of oil, use 6 teaspoons (2 tablespoons), and you'll cut the fat by half.

- Use broth and/or wine as a substitute for oil when sautéeing or stir-frying. Be sure to cook over a high heat and add just enough liquid to keep your veggies/meat from sticking or burning. Continue to slowly add liquid until they are cooked to your liking.

- You can make the best french fries by placing potato strips in a zip-lock baggie with 2 tablespoons of oil

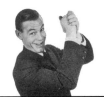

and your favorite seasonings. Shake it up until the potatoes are well coated, then bake them at 400 degrees, turning them every seven minutes until they are golden brown and crispy.

- Replace the oil in marinade recipes with plain seltzer water. You'll get the same results without the fat— tender meat and lots of flavor.

- Switch to 'unfrying' your chicken or fish. Use egg whites or yogurt to help the bread crumbs or corn flakes adhere to the meat (if you choose yogurt, make sure it is very cold, and soak your meat in ice water before dipping it in the yogurt). Instead of deep frying, you can bake them in the oven with just a few sprays of oil.

- When a recipe requires browning the meat, do it under the broiler rather then in a pan with oil. Coat it with flour and place it in a shallow baking pan. Broil, stirring it occasionally until it is browned on all sides. Then remove it from the pan with a slotted spoon.

- Create thick and creamy soups without adding fat. Purée half of the soup in a blender and then add it back to the remaining soup. Or, you can add puréed potatoes or cannellini beans as thickeners.

- Enhance the flavor of your foods with herbs and spices. Use fresh herbs in place of dried, increasing the amount three-fold.

- Always use the freshest and best ingredients. That means crushing your own garlic, squeezing real

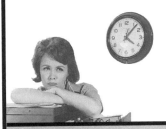

A COMPLETE WASTE OF TIME

The 3 Worst Things You Can Do When It Comes to Preparing Your Food Are:

1. Fry everything.
2. Don't look for fat alternatives.
3. Rely on prepackaged foods.

lemons or limes for their juice, grating nutmeg and ginger, grinding pepper, using pure vanilla extract, and cooking with the best seasonal produce available. You can choose from a variety of flavor boosters listed in Chapter 2, "Supplies and Equipment Worth Their Weight" ("Pinch an Inch for Size, Add a Dash for Taste").

Deserting the Fat but Not Your Desserts

It's hard to think of living without desserts, so don't. But you can easily dream of having delicious desserts without all of the fat, especially when you follow these tips.

- You should never remove all of the fat in your baked goods, but you can get rid of some. For instance, if your recipe calls for $1/2$ cup, try using $1/3$ cup. Keep experimenting with lowering the fat until you can have the taste and texture you desire with the least amount of fat.

- Replace all eggs with egg substitute ($1/4$ cup = 1 egg), egg whites (1 large egg white + 1 teaspoon water = 1 egg), or a combination of both. If you are making custard or need a tender, flaky texture, reduce the number of egg yolks rather than replacing all of them.

- Always replace whole milk with skim milk. Canned evaporated skim milk has a slightly thicker texture and sweeter taste.

- Use fruit purées (applesauce, bananas, prunes, pumpkin) to replace half of the butter or margarine

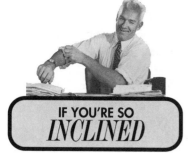

IF YOU'RE SO
INCLINED

Fill up with flavor not with fat. Day-old bread works at the bakery, but fresh is best when you're using herbs and spices. The closer it is to the source, the more intense your flavor will be. Go ahead and zest your lemons, grate your ginger, and crush your garlic!

in a recipe. Prune purées are especially good with chocolate items. You can also use nonfat yogurt, sour cream, or buttermilk.

- When a recipe calls for unsweetened chocolate bars (baker's chocolate), substitute unsweetened cocoa powder for half of the bars. Use 2 heaping table-spoons for every ounce of unsweetened chocolate removed.

- Use mini chocolate chips instead of regular size ones. This way you can cut back on the amount you use and still get an even distribution of chocolate throughout the dessert.

- Decrease the amount of nuts you use or omit them altogether. You can intensify their flavor by lightly toasting them in a 350-degree oven. Let them cool completely, then chop them up finely for maximum distribution.

- Always use pure vanilla extract in your recipes. Adding a little more of this flavoring can enhance the sweetness of your dessert. Other flavor boosters are brandy, coffee, liqueurs, almond extract, and molasses.

- To cut back on calories, decrease the amount of sugar by half. You won't miss it a bit.

FILL-INS THAT WON'T FILL YOU UP

You may wonder if it's worth altering certain foods that are oozing with fat. After all, if you get rid of the fat, you

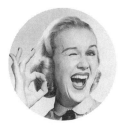

Try it. You'll like it! These days just about every condiment available has a low fat or nonfat cousin. Explore your condiment's family tree by trying and buying the low fat or nonfat versions of mayonnaise, sour cream, cream cheese, and salad dressings. If you replace your existing brands with their low fat relatives, you'll save time, energy, and fat.

take away the reason why we eat them—their rich, creamy taste and texture. But you can make a few simple changes and not even know the difference (except in your dwindling waistline). Here are some delicious substitutes for dressings, sauces, ice cream, and cream cheese.

Dressings

Here's how to dress (your veggies and sandwiches) for pound shedding success.

- Recipes using regular mayonnaise and dairy products as their creamy base can be replaced with the nonfat versions of these ingredients. For example, blend a mixture of nonfat sour cream (or mayonnaise) and skim milk with your salad dressing seasoning packet. Enhance the flavor by adding your favorite fresh herbs.

- Switch the ratio for your oil and vinegar dressings. Instead of three parts oil to one part vinegar, use three parts vinegar to one part oil. Try different flavored vinegars. Some of them are good enough to use without the oil.

- Make some skinny sandwich spreads by combining nonfat mayonnaise with dijon-style mustard, horse radish, minced onion, or garlic and/or fresh herbs. These spreads can also dress up your artichokes or asparagus.

Sauces

How about sauces that are sassy instead of fatty?

- You can still enjoy a creamy sauce by using a little less butter for your roux and then substituting skim milk for cream. If your sauce is lumpy, blend it in the cuisinart for a minute or two. Adding a little nonfat sour cream will enhance the richness of this sauce.

- Create a cheesy sauce from the one above by adding a small amount of intensely flavored cheese such as sharp cheddar, parmesan, or peppered jack. A little bit of flavor goes a lot further.

- You can make your own half and half by blending $1/2$ cup buttermilk with $1/2$ cup nonfat vanilla yogurt.

- Give salsas and chutney a try. They are a delicious substitute for heavy sauces.

Ice Cream

These low fat alternatives will make you forget that you ever screamed for ice cream.

- Switch from regular ice cream to a nonfat/low fat variety, ice milk, or nonfat frozen yogurt. Read labels to make sure you don't go overboard on calories.

- Try a fruit sorbet or glace. Their intense flavor keeps you from over indulging.

- Don't forget pudding pops. You can get the same satisfaction of licking an ice cream cone without a lot of fat.

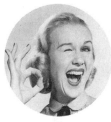

QUICK 🆔 PAINLESS

You deserve a shake today. But make sure you "moo"ve on over to low fat or nonfat varieties. The taste will still be great, and you'll be significantly decreasing your fat intake. It does your body (and soul) good.

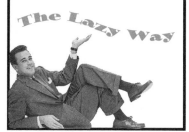
Cream Cheese

Can it be not as creamy, but just as dreamy? You bet!

- Switch to the low fat or nonfat versions of cream cheese. When using nonfat cream cheese in baking, add 1 tablespoon of cornstarch per 8 ounces of cream cheese to keep it from separating.

- You can substitute half of your cream cheese with nonfat ricotta or sour cream.

- Here's a delicious fill-in for a creamy cheese filling that you can use in crepes, blintzes, or cheesecakes:

  1. Combine 2 cups low fat (1%) cottage cheese with 1 tablespoon sugar and purée until thick and creamy.

  2. Stir in 1 teaspoon pure vanilla extract.

  3. Pour the mixture into a yogurt strainer or a sieve lined with cheesecloth, and place this over a bowl to catch the drippings.

  4. Refrigerate for 20 to 24 hours. Discard drippings. Store in a sealed container in the refrigerator until ready to use (for up to a week).

CAN YOU BELIEVE IT'S NOT BUTTER?!

We don't expect you to waste time churning back and forth from butter to margarine (and vice versa) every time a new study comes out claiming one or the other is the 'bad guy.' Just make it easy on yourself and stick to the real thing—butter! You're only going to have a pat or two anyway, so why not enjoy the natural stuff?

If you are concerned about your cholesterol intake, you may decide to use margarine over butter (margarine is derived from plant oil, so it has no cholesterol). If that's the case, be sure to choose margarines that are only partially hydrogenated such as margarine sprays, canola, or 'trans-free' spreads.

Butter is now being molded into different products with a lot less fat. Light butter (made with skim milk) and yogurt butter (blended with yogurt) have less than half the calories and fat grams of whole butter. You can also use whipped butter to lighten your fat load. Butter flakes are a great substitute for sprinkling on popcorn, mashed potatoes, and steamed veggies. Be sure to try these products to see which ones you like the best.

When you focus on cutting back the fat, you are taking a shortcut to shedding the pounds permanently. The more you can do this with your daily meals, the better off you'll be. But what about those favorite treats that just aren't worth eating without the fat? You can still have your goodies (and eat them too!) if you practice a little portion control. We'll tell you all about it in the next chapter.

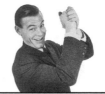

YOU'LL THANK YOURSELF LATER

One pat or two? If you're having a hard time estimating the amount of butter you can spread on your low fat bagel or toast, buy the prewrapped restaurant style instead. After reading the fat content on the label, you'll know effortlessly whether you can have one pat or two.

Getting Time on Your Side

	The Old Way	The Lazy Way
Searching for the fat	10 minutes	2 minutes
Using substitutions instead of fat	10 minutes	2 minutes
Trimming the fat	5 minutes	1 minute
Modifying recipes	40 minutes	2 minutes
Decreasing calories	20 minutes	3 minutes
Missing the fat	Every day	Never again!

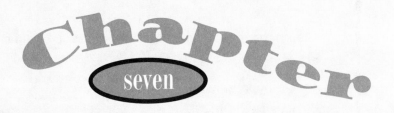

Divide and Devour

Super Sizes . . . Big Gulps . . . Double Deckers . . . The dimensions available these days are designed for the land of the giants (and giants we shall become). Bigger is not better when it embodies portion size. Don't forget that good things can come in small packages too.

In this chapter we'll show you the effortless system of parceling your goods. You'll know how to size up your servings and downsize your treats. You'll be given a free rein on free foods. And, you'll get the scoop on how the right portions can lead to the proper proportions.

SIZING UP YOUR SERVINGS IN SECONDS

Figuring your portions *The Lazy Way* does not require any exact measurements or weights. It just takes your eyeballs and a little practice. Make it easy on yourself and swap measurements with common objects pictured in your mind like balls, dominoes, and bottle caps.

These comparisons will help you get a handle on your portions.

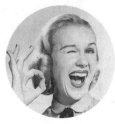

QUICK **n** PAINLESS

The eyes have it! Serving size shouldn't leave you serving time at the gym. Be able to recognize at a glance (or in a gulp) how much you can (or did) consume.

- 1 teaspoon is about the size of a bottle cap or a pat of butter.

- 1 tablespoon is about the size of an ice cube.

- $1/4$ cup is about the size of a large egg.

- $1/2$ cup is about the size of a racquetball.

- $3/4$ cup is about the size of a tennis ball.

- 1 cup is about the size of a baseball or your clenched fist.

- 1 ounce is about the size of a domino.

- 3 ounces is about the size of your palm (minus your fingers) or a deck of playing cards.

Now you can easily size up your portions of the different food groups. Remember that you want to eat mostly wholesome grains and starches, legumes, and vegetables. Eat moderate amounts of fruit and small amounts of dairy, meat, eggs, cheese, and nuts. Last, and it is the least, eat fats and sugars sparingly.

Here's a simple guideline that breaks down your servings:

- Six to 11 servings of breads, cereals, legumes*, and grains.

  A serving of grain foods—bread, cereal, rice, and pasta—is equal to one slice of bread, $1/2$ an English muffin or small bagel, $1/2$ cup of cooked grains (rice, pasta, barley, etc.), and $3/4$ cup ready-to-eat cereal. A serving of your legumes equals $1/2$ cup.

- Four to six servings of vegetables.

  A serving of vegetables is equal to $1/2$ cup of regular veggies or 1 cup of leafy greens.

- Two to four servings of fruit.

  A serving of fruit is considered one medium whole fruit (tennis ball), $1/2$ cup of cut-up fruit, or $3/4$ cup of juice.

- Two servings of dairy.

  A serving of dairy is equal to 1 cup of most nonfat dairy products (milk, yogurt, cottage cheese) and $1/2$ cup of nonfat frozen yogurt.

- Two servings (4 to 6 ounces) of meats, eggs, legumes*, and cheese.

  A serving of meat, fish, and poultry is 3 ounces cooked. A serving of cheese is 1 ounce. Eggs and legumes count as 1 ounce of meat (one egg and $1/2$ cup beans).

- Two to three servings of fat.

  A serving of fat is equal to 1 teaspoon.

- Eight to 15 servings of (added) sugar.

  A serving of sugar is equal to 1 teaspoon.

  * $1/2$ cup of legumes or beans is equal to one serving of the grain foods AND 1 ounce of meat.

HAVE A FULL PLATE WITHOUT FEELING FULL

Now that you have an idea of how much you get to eat, you can mix and match your food servings for your meals

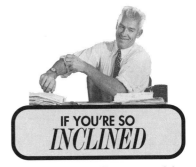

IF YOU'RE SO
INCLINED

Plant a small vegetable garden with some of your favorite produce. You won't have to run to the market every time you need veggies, and it will taste all the sweeter (and more flavorful) knowing it was organically grown in your own backyard.

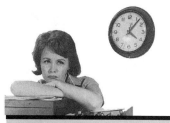

The 3 Worst Things You Can Do When It Comes to Creating a Meal Are:

1. Don't create a balanced plate.

2. Overdo your portions.

3. Eat more than you need (you can always save it for later!).

throughout the day. We'll show you how simple it is to create your breakfasts, lunches, and dinners (don't forget snacks and desserts) using the different food groups. But, first let's look at a few rules before filling up your plate.

When you think of the portions on your plate, keep in mind that $3/4$ of your food should be a combination of grains/legumes, vegetables, or fruits. The other $1/4$ should be your protein (meat, eggs, cheese, or nuts). Never have more than two to three servings of the grain foods (breads, cereal, rice, and pasta) at one meal. Finally, eat no more that 2 to $2^1/2$ cups of food at one sitting.

A serving from here, a serving from there . . . now all you need is your silverware.

- A mixture of grain foods with some dairy and fruit will give you a high-energy breakfast to start you off in the morning. Two grains plus two fruits and a serving of dairy could be $1^1/2$ cups ready-to-eat cereal with 1 cup of nonfat milk and a banana OR two pieces of whole-wheat toast with all-fruit jam (2 tablespoons), 1 cup of nonfat yogurt, and 6 ounces of orange juice.

- A serving of your favorite fruit makes a great mid-morning snack. You can choose an apple, orange, or peach if you'd like, just make sure it's the size of a tennis ball.

- Fill your lunch sack with a combination of grains (2), proteins (1), veggies (2), and a serving of fat (1). You could have a turkey sandwich made with 1 tablespoon of low fat mayo and two handfuls of carrot sticks OR you could opt for a salad with low fat dressing followed by a bean burrito with 1 ounce of low fat cheese.

- Have a wholesome grain and a fruit or vegetable to pick you up in the afternoon. You could snack on two graham cracker rectangles, 3 cups of light popcorn, or a handful of whole wheat pretzels along with 6 ounces of V-8 juice or a few pieces of dried fruit.

- Dinner is probably the meal at which you get the most of your servings at one sitting. You can keep it balanced by choosing three grains, three veggies, and a protein topped with a serving of fat (usually used in preparing the meal). You could serve up spaghetti (1 to $1^1/2$ cup pasta with $^1/2$ cup tomato sauce) with meat balls (2 to 3 ounces) and 1 cup of steamed veggies OR a chicken breast stir-fried with veggies ($1^1/2$ cup) and teriyaki sauce over rice (1 to $1^1/2$ cup).

- You can end your evening with a serving of dairy for dessert. Nonfat frozen yogurt or sherbet ($^1/2$ cup), a fudgsicle, or a cup of nonfat cocoa are some of the choices you can make for this food group.

So, these are just some of the ways you can mix and match your food servings to create your meals. It's quite simple once you know what a portion is. And when you watch your portions, your eyes will grant you a smaller stomach.

Congratulations! You've watched your portions for a week! Take a break and go see a movie with your family!

The Lazy Way

Long division with a remainder of none. Parcel out your week's worth of snacks once a week. Divvy up a daily serving of each of the five food groups into individual zippered bags and place each day's worth into one larger zippered bag. You'll meet your minimum daily requirement without a week's worth of thought.

TIPS FOR DOWNSIZING YOUR TREATS

There are some rich morsels that just wouldn't cut it if you cut the fat. And, we would never expect you to give them up. The plan of attack is simple—divvy them up into mini-morsels.

The following tips will get you ready to divide and devour.

- Read the food labels of all your treats. Decrease the serving size until your portion contains no more than 75 calories and 2 grams of fat.

- You don't have to desert Mrs. Field's cookies. Buy the frozen variety, and cut each cookie into quarters before baking.

- Monitor your M&Ms. Instead of gobbling a handful (50 pieces = 220 calories and 9 grams of fat), give yourself two of each color (brown, blue, red, green, orange, and yellow), (12 pieces = 60 calories and 2 grams of fat).

- Always choose the mini-sized candy bars. If you buy a bag of them, keep it on the highest shelf of your snack cupboard. When you want a candy bar, take one piece from the bag and seal it back up and close your cupboard.

- When a recipe (brownie, cake, pie, etc.) gives you the number of servings it will divide into, go ahead and divide them again. A smaller piece will save you half the fat and calories.

- When you're in front of a buffet table brimming with delectable delicacies, make sure you use the smallest plate and take just a bite of the three items most appealing to you.

- Another way to have your cake and eat it is to trade food calories for exercise ones. Check out the chart on page 150 to figure out what you need to do to burn off your favorite treats.

So, there's no need to deprive yourself. Go ahead and splurge if you get the urge—it just has to be a mini one.

FREE REIN ON FREE FOODS

You can consume a number of foods without fretting too much about their portion size. These foods are considered 'free' because they have minimal calories and maybe just a trace of fat. Of course, if you have a gallon of one or a pound of the other, they'll end up being a burden. But, we know you won't do that—after all, huge amounts would take too much time to eat.

You can loosen the reins on the following free foods:

- Butter flakes
- Celery
- Chile peppers
- Club soda
- Dill pickles (small)
- Flavoring extracts (almond, vanilla, etc.)
- Garlic
- Gelatin (unflavored or sugar-free/low calorie)*
- Herbal teas
- Herbs and spices

If you've been slavin' away around the bottom of the food pyramid then don't de"Nile" yourself any longer. Act like royalty and savor a single sweet from the top.

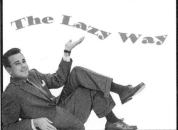

The Lazy Way

- Horse radish
- Leafy greens
- Lemon/lime juice
- Mustard
- Onions
- Pimiento
- Soy sauce (light sodium)
- Sugar-free gum/mints (up to five a day)*
- Sugar-free soft drinks*
- Sugar substitutes (aspartame, saccharin, etc.)*
- Tonic water (sugar-free)*
- Vinegar
- Water (plain, mineral, or carbonated)
- Wine used in cooking
- Worcestershire sauce

*Although sugar substitutes do help you avoid sugar calories in the short run, their use doesn't decrease your overall desire for sweets. By reducing all sweeteners, your taste buds gradually adjust so that less sweet foods taste sweeter.

Vegetables are another food you can veg out on. They're a great source of vitamins, minerals, and fiber, plus, they just have a trace of fat! (That is unless you add butter, mayonnaise, or oil.) So, go ahead, indulge yourself, and freeload on the veggies.

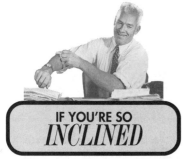

IF YOU'RE SO
INCLINED

Here's a fast pitch for your speedy meal planning. Large, medium, and small—it's the perfect batting order for your eating needs. The line up: breakfast, your largest meal; add a medium repast at lunch; and, top it off with a light supper.

Watching what you eat by eyeing your portions is so simple. You won't get blurred vision examining calorie charts or scale meters. And, if you take the time to figure out your appropriate servings, you'll enjoy the time spent by the mirror gazing at your figure.

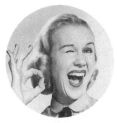

QUICK n' PAINLESS

No more calorie counting! Eye your portions and watch yourself shed some pounds effortlessly!

Getting Time on Your Side

	The Old Way	The Lazy Way
Selecting treats	10 minutes	3 minutes
Weighing your food	5 minutes	In a blink (0 minutes)
Measuring your food	3 minutes	In a wink (0 minutes)
Eating tasteless "diet food"	Years	Never again
Sizing up your portions	Hours	2 seconds
Keeping your snacking under control	Impossible!	15 minutes, once a week

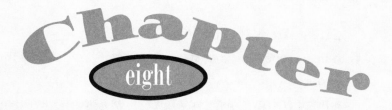

To Spread or to Shed?

The weight loss industry is bursting at the seams with pills, powders, and potions. That's because we all want a fast and easy way to lose the pounds. But, when you rely on these panaceas, the only thing you lose is time and money. Kind of hard to swallow, huh?

Well, here's some news that will go down smoothly. There are some tricks of the diet trade that have been proven to help you shed the pounds effortlessly. And, you don't have to spend a dime. Let these tried and true tips assist you in avoiding the spread and boosting the shed.

FAT SPREADERS

Besides overindulging in plain ol' fat, there are other aspects of eating that can cause you to spread. They include starving yourself, drinking alcoholic beverages, overdosing on sugars, and eating late at night. Here's why you should give up these habits.

Starvation Is Not Your Salvation

It bears repeating that starving yourself is absolutely the wrong way to shed some pounds. Not only is deprivation a huge energy drain—you have to exercise extreme will power to keep food from passing through the lips (mentally and perhaps manually)—it causes your body to work extra hard at providing itself with energy. The only thing that comes easy is the (wide) spreading of fat!

If you want to refresh your memory on how starvation backfires on you, just review the "Don't Bother Fasting; It Isn't Very Lasting" section of Chapter 1.

You Lose Your Leverage with an Alcoholic Beverage

Next to fat, alcohol has the second highest amount of calories per gram (1 gram of fat = 9 calories/1 gram of alcohol = 7 calories). An average drink contains anywhere from 100 to 160 calories. This is the primary reason why alcohol is considered a fat spreader, but there are other factors that cause it to be tipsy on your scale. The following list may help encourage you to boo the booze.

- Alcohol is a depressant. Not only will it slow down brain activity, it will decrease your metabolism too.

- This drug provides no essential nutrients, and it actually depletes every nutrient in your body to some extent.

- When calories from alcohol are not used as an immediate source of energy, they are quickly converted to fat, ready to be stored.

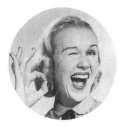

- Alcohol is a diuretic. It drains valuable water, vitamins, and minerals from your body.

- Imbibing increases your appetite. Coupling this with a lowered inhibition can lead you to over indulge.

- Drinking too much alcohol can leave you feeling lethargic. This diminishes your energy and enthusiasm when it comes to working out.

De Agony of De Sweet

When refined sugar was first introduced, the average American consumption was around 5 pounds a year. Now, as we journey into the 21st century, the annual consumption of these sweet granules is over 130 pounds. That means we go through the equivalent of a 5-pound bag every two weeks! (Most of which comes from packaged, processed food products.)

Eating excess amounts of refined sugar can spread the fat like icing on a cake. And, it's not just the white stuff . . . refined sugars also include brown sugar, raw sugar, corn syrup, honey, molasses, and refined white flours (i.e., white bread, rice, pretzels, and packaged pastas). These sugars break down quickly in your blood stream, and if you eat large amounts they will raise your blood sugar (glucose) to abnormal levels. Your body will react by releasing insulin, which tries to return your blood sugar to a normal level. If your muscles cannot absorb all of the sugar, insulin will convert any excess sugar to fat! The bad news is your body cannot convert

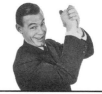

YOU'LL THANK YOURSELF LATER

What's your alcoholic beverage of choice? Find out the caloric content of your favorite cocktail. Try to substitute a lighter version of the real thing to cut back on calories without compromising flavor. Next time the cocktail hour strikes try this instead:

1. Order a light or non-alcoholic version of your favorite beer or wine.

2. Order your favorite cocktail in a tall glass with more ice or water added.

3. Order a Virgin Bloody Mary.

the fat back to sugar. The only way to get rid of the fat is to burn it off with exercise.

Another problem with refined sugars is that they have little nutritional value. They don't signal the brain that you are full and the continual spiking of blood sugar can cause you to crave more sweets.

So, don't overdo the sugar. Try to keep your refined sugar intake around 8 to 15 teaspoons a day. (See Chapter 4 to determine how much sugar is in a food product.) Here is a list of foods that tend to be loaded with the sweet stuff (sugar content is approximate per average serving).

- Cake (8 teaspoons)
- Canned fruit in heavy syrup (9 teaspoons)
- Cereal (4 teaspoons)
- Chocolate milk (4 teaspoons)
- Cookies (3 teaspoons)
- Doughnuts, glazed (7$\frac{1}{2}$ teaspoons)
- Energy bars (4 teaspoons)
- Granola bars (3 teaspoons)
- Hard candy (5 teaspoons)
- Ice cream (6$\frac{1}{2}$ teaspoons)
- Jams/jellies (3$\frac{1}{2}$ teaspoons)
- Pie (10 teaspoons)
- Soft drinks (9 teaspoons)
- Sweetened yogurts (8 teaspoons)

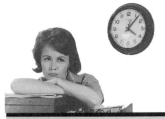

A COMPLETE WASTE OF TIME

The 3 Worst Things You Can Do When It Comes to Sugar Are:

1. Overdo it.

2. Forget to see how much refined sugar is in the food you eat.

3. Think that sugars have nutritional value.

Midnight Munchies Leave Your Bedsheet Crunchy and Your Jeans All Bunchy

Eating late at night spreads more than crumbs on your couch or bed. The reason why this nocturnal activity plumps you up is because your metabolism is winding down to its lowest point (sleeping). Your body and brain need the most energy during the first half of your day. This is when your metabolism and body temperature are at their highest levels. It is during this time that you should get most of your fuel (food) in.

Once the majority of your waking hours are over, your body needs less energy—it decreases the amount of calories it burns. That's why it's important to start cutting back at dinner time. Unfortunately, most of us tend to have our biggest meal in the evening. When you do this, you are not matching your eating to your metabolism. You take yourself even further off track when you continue eating late into the night.

So, try to lighten your supper and make it a rule not to eat less than two to three hours before bedtime. This is a healthy habit that will help you be more successful at losing weight and keeping it off. Remind yourself that daytime calories are easily burned and nighttime calories are easily stored.

FAT SHEDDERS

We're sorry we can't recommend a pill or potion to melt the fat away. However, there are still effortless ways to shed the fat without any side effects. You can start by eating a wholesome breakfast and continuing to eat

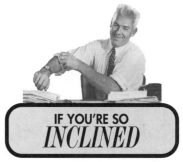

IF YOU'RE SO
INCLINED

Does your appetite kick in when the late show ends? If you're an incurable late snacker, try this tip to help avoid adding pounds as you're counting sheep. Plan to have a low fat snack during the early evening then drink a glass of water before you climb between the sheets.

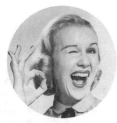

small meals all day long. Add some water and spice and you'll be shedding in no time.

Grazing Is Udderly Amazing

Your body is designed to eat small meals frequently throughout the day. This helps it to:

- Keep your blood sugar constant.
- Keep your energy levels elevated.
- Readily burn calories.
- Maintain a good mood.
- Suppress your appetite.
- Be reassured that it will get the energy it needs.

When you eat five to six small meals a day (the smallest of them at night), you are maximizing your body's fat shedding power. Therefore, never go more than three to four hours without having something to eat.

Wada! Wada! Wada!

Perhaps you've already heard about the importance of drinking your water. They've told you it's good for this, it's good for that—yada, yada, yada . . . But, did you know water also helps your body shed the pounds?

Water is necessary for every single function of every single cell in your body. This includes the reaction that releases fat from your fat cells. When you drink enough water, your body can function at its best, keeping you balanced and healthy. This ensures that your digestion and metabolism are working at full capacity. Water also enhances your performance when you exercise, keeping your muscles cooled and flushed, thereby preventing fatigue.

This wonder tonic is the key to unlocking the extra weight of fluid retention. Water retention from hormones and excess salt can be eliminated by drinking more water. Water stored in extra cellular space (outside the cells) can cause your feet, hands, legs, and abdomen to swell. Drinking water will help release stored fluid and get rid of excess sodium. It will also counteract the dehydrating effect of caffeine and alcohol, which slows down fat loss.

There's no doubt that drinking enough water will help boost your fat shedding. The clouded part comes in trying to meet your water quota. These drops of advice will have you filling up with this miraculous fluid in no time.

- Your body loses water gradually throughout the day, so it's best to take it in gradually.

- Try to begin your morning with a glass of pure water. Then drink a glass with every meal and every time you brush your teeth (rinse first!).

- Give your plain water some pizzazz with a squeeze of lemon, a sprig of mint, or a splash of low calorie cranberry juice.

- Make it a habit to carry a water bottle around with you.

- Select juicy fruits like peaches, strawberries, and watermelon. These fruits, along with most veggies, have a high water content.

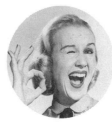

QUICK ⬤ PAINLESS

Water, water, water! It's good for you, it curbs those snack attacks— what more could you want from a beverage? Have some!

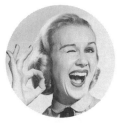

- Avoid caffinated beverages—switch to herbal teas.

- Drink your water ice cold for a metabolic boost. Your body will burn a few extra calories in warming up the water to normal body temperature.

Sprinkle Some Spice and the Calories Melt Like Ice

Just as ice cold water boosts your metabolism, adding a little hot stuff will give you the same effect. This effect is called thermogenesis—the amount of calories burned digesting, absorbing, and utilizing food. Some foods have a higher thermic effect, the most notable ones being hot peppers and mustard.

So, give spicy foods a try. Start adding some sizzle to your stir-fries, soups, stews, salsas, and spreads. Here's a list of hot stuff that will spice up your meals and metabolism.

- Cayenne pepper
- Dried hot pepper flakes
- Horseradish
- Hot chile peppers (habañero, jalapeño, serrano)
- Hot mustard
- Hot paprika
- Hot sauce
- Mustard seeds
- Spicy salsas
- Wasabi

Break the Fast with Breakfast

Yes, it's true . . . breakfast is your most important meal. It is the first fuel you give your body for the day. Skipping breakfast may cause your blood sugar level to drop below normal, resulting in fatigue, headaches, weakness, and loss of concentration. A good breakfast improves your mental and physical performance, gives you energy, and reduces your hunger during the morning.

You may have skipped breakfast in the past due to lack of time or an appetite. But, now that you know this first meal has such an impact on your energy, you won't want to miss it. Here are some quick-fix breakfast ideas that can help you make a fast break into becoming a better fat shedder.

- Stock up your refrigerator with nonfat yogurt. It's great by itself or you can add some Grape Nuts or fresh fruit. Use it on your pancakes instead of syrup. Or, you can toss it in the blender with some frozen fruit chunks to make a quick smoothie.

- Make your own packets of quick oatmeal by putting some quick-cooking oats, cinnamon, and raisins (or any dried fruit) in sealed baggies. You'll just need to add hot water and a sprinkle of brown sugar.

- Buy whole-grain frozen waffles. Just pop them in the toaster and you're off.

- Have two or three wholesome cereals that you can choose from during the week.

- Heat up leftovers.

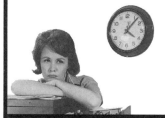

A COMPLETE WASTE OF TIME

The 3 Worst Effects of Skipping Breakfast:

1. You'll be more hungry much sooner.

2. You'll tire more quickly.

3. You'll be unable to work as effectively/ efficiently.

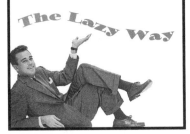
▨ Put a slice of tofu cheese or mozzarella on a piece of whole wheat bread, add a tomato if you like, and place it under the broiler.

▨ Make (or order) a healthy egg muffin. Skip the butter and cheese and you drastically lower the fat and calories.

Well, there you have it. No hype or empty promises, just the facts on how your body can either spread or shed the fat. So, forget about the fasting or munching at midnight. Lose the booze and skip the sugar. Remember to start each day with breakfast. Eat frequent, small, spicy meals, and drink them down with lots of water. You'll be shedding your fat in no time.

Getting Time on Your Side

	The Old Way	**The Lazy Way**
Starving yourself	24 hours	Never
Savoring sweets	10 minutes	0 minutes
Selecting cocktails	5 minutes	2 minutes
Craving that midnight snack	Every night	Never again!
Getting the munchies	All day	Never
Staying focused in the morning	Impossible!	Always! (now that you eat breakfast!)

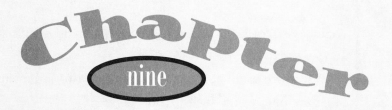

Dining on the Dash

You are the last car in line, and you vacillate between staying there or parking and placing your order inside. You're not sure which will be faster, but you decide to stick to the drive-thru since you're already there anyway. After a few minutes of idling, you trade money for food and you're on your way. Sound familiar?

It seems the busier we get, the more we depend on drive-thrus, restaurants, vending machines, and prepared meals for our daily nourishment. Relying on these sources may save us time, yet they can also preserve our poundage (and then some). Now, we don't expect you to give up this convenient mode of consumption, but there are some rules you should follow to steer you in the right direction.

FAST FOOD—YOU DON'T HAVE TO FAST

The good news is, fast food restaurants are not off-limits. You can order a meal at any of these joints without blowing your fat budget. Of course, we're not talking about a double-decker burger with a giant order of fries (that could be two days' worth of fat). We mean choosing a menu item that is low in fat.

Here are some pointers for selecting fast food meals that are happy and healthy too.

- Most fast food restaurants use regular processed cheese which is high in fat and calories. Get in the habit of omitting the cheese from any item that you order.

- Order your muffins, biscuits, or sandwiches without any butter, mayonnaise, or mayonnaise-based sauces.

- Choose a broiled chicken sandwich over a hamburger or a breaded, deep-fried chicken/fish sandwich.

- Avoid the deluxe or jumbo versions of any menu items. Always choose the smallest size offered (it's usually regular).

- If fried chicken is your only choice, choose the regular coating over the extra crispy type and make sure you peel the skin off.

- When selecting a pizza, opt for a thin crust and tell them to go easy on the cheese. If you add an extra topping make sure it's veggies (but tell them to hold the olives).

- If a fast food restaurant offers potatoes, order yours plain.

- Consult the fast food nutrition guides to find out if your favorite menu items are healthy. Try to keep your fast food meal around 500 to 600 calories and 12 to 18 grams of fat.

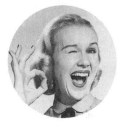

QUICK ☞ PAINLESS

Do you need that side of fries with your meal, or do you order it out of habit? Try skipping it next time you drive-thru and see if you miss it. You could always bring along an apple instead!

OUT TO LUNCH (OR ANY MEAL FOR THAT MATTER)

Dining out can be a daunting experience when you are trying to shed some pounds. You know how it is . . . you're tempted by the dessert tray practically the minute you walk into the place, you're never quite sure how much fat the chef uses behind closed doors, and virtually everything on the menu sounds enticing.

This wouldn't be such a problem if you dined out once or twice a month—you could have whatever your heart desires (they probably won't let you buy the whole dessert cart). But, if you eat more than two or three meals a week in restaurants, you need to be more selective.

Here are some tips to help you dine out without a dash of concern.

- Try to restrict alcoholic drinks. Alcohol is not only loaded with empty calories, but it can increase your appetite and decrease your self-control. Choose a wine spritzer, lite or nonalcoholic beer, or a Virgin Bloody Mary. Always ask for a glass of water as soon as you're seated.

- Limit yourself to one piece of bread and/or one handful of chips.

- Appetizers can be on both sides of the fat fence. Stay away from items that are deep-fried or full of cheese. Gravitate toward consommés, soups, vegetable platters, or shrimp cocktails.

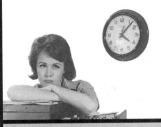

A COMPLETE WASTE OF TIME

The 3 Worst Effects of Ordering Alcoholic Beverages When You're Eating Out:

1. Increases your load of empty calories.

2. Increases your appetite.

3. Decreases your self-control.

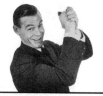

As your eyes meander over the menu, keep this in mind: The four healthiest ways to have your food prepared are baked, broiled, grilled, or poached.

■ Ordering two appetizers instead of an entree can help you keep your portion sizes small.

■ When at the salad bar, fill your plate with lots of raw veggies, and pass on the prepared salads like potato, pasta, or oil-marinated veggies. Use seeds, croutons, bacon bits, and hard boiled eggs sparingly.

■ Always ask for your dressing and sauces on the side. Then you can dip your fork in them to get a little flavor with each bite.

■ The healthiest ways for the chef to prepare your main dish (chicken, fish, or meat) are baked, broiled, grilled (no butter), or poached.

■ Avoid menu items that contain words like scalloped, deep fried, au gratin, béarnaise, or hollandaise sauce.

■ If you must succumb to the dessert tray, choose items like fresh fruit, sorbets, or angel food cake. Share your dessert with your companion(s).

■ When ordering your mocha or latte be sure to ask for nonfat milk. You won't miss a thing with this request except for fat and calories.

GOING OUT BUT NOT OUT OF CONTROL

Some of the hardest times to make healthy food choices are when you are invited out to parties, weddings, and other social functions . . . mostly because you have to look pretty hard to find some morsels that haven't been drowned in fat and calories (other than the boring crudités tray). But, there is a way to indulge without losing control. You just need to plan your course of action.

These simple strategies will keep you on course:

- The best way to handle food in social situations is to take small (maybe even tiny) amounts of what's offered.

- At a party buffet, if they offer a choice of plate size, use the smaller one. Pass on any refills.

- Try to stay away from the hors d'oeuvres table(s). Focus your attention on the company and audience rather than just the food.

- Avoid alcohol and choose no-calorie beverages instead. Try a glass of seltzer with cranberry juice and a squeeze of lime or a nonalcoholic beer.

- When you know you're going to be eating rich foods that night, choose to eat healthy low fat meals during the day. Be sure that you aren't starving when you go out, though—this could make you overindulge. Have a light snack before you go out to take the edge off your appetite.

- You can always stick to the crudités tray if you want to be extra good.

- Whenever there's dancing, be sure you bring your boogie shoes to burn up the extra calories.

THE WORK DAY GRUB

It usually happens between 2:30 and 3:00 in the afternoon . . . your stomach and/or your brain (you're not sure which one) decides you are hungry and leaves you in a

Congratulations! You made low fat choices all day long, so go ahead and splurge a little at your social function.

The Lazy Way

state of rumbling and grumbling. You nod off, hoping this may quiet them down, only to dream that the candy bars in the vending machine are fighting over which one will be next to take the big plunge. Of course, they want you to pick the winner . . .

This is just one of the scenarios you may toil with at work. Eating healthy on the job can be a labored process. It could be a matter of not having enough time or even having too much. Or, it may be those tempting morsels hanging out amongst your memos.

Here are some ways to keep the work day grub healthy without making it a chore.

- It's best to steer clear of vending machines. If you're hungry, chances are you'll think all of the candy bars should be winners. Most items in the vending machines are losers when it comes to being low in fat, calories, sugar, and sodium.

- Stock your desk with low fat snacks at the beginning of each week.

- Keep a bottle of water at your desk and drink from it throughout the day.

- If you know you are going to be spending your lunch hour at work, try and prepare a healthy meal the night before. This will keep you from skipping lunch or going out for more fattening fare.

- Skip the doughnuts, croissants, and muffins at those breakfast meetings—they're loaded with fat and calories. Choose some fruit, fruit juice, or a bagel instead.

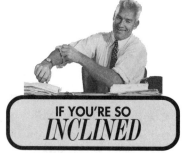

IF YOU'RE SO
INCLINED

Make your snacks at home so you know they're healthy, and carry them with you so you'll be prepared for those annoying snack attacks!

HOW TO DEAL WITH THAT PREPARED MEAL

We just don't have the time or desire to spend more than half an hour in the kitchen these days. So, most of us rely on prepackaged or prepared foods to help us create a home-cooked meal in a jiffy. Sometimes we're so quick, all we have to do is heat it up!

The dilemma is, how do you eat real, wholesome, low fat food when it comes out of a box? The following cartes du jour will show you how to deal with that prepared meal.

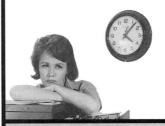

A COMPLETE WASTE OF TIME

The 3 Worst Items to Find High Levels of Listed in the Nutritional Label on Your Prepared Meal Container:

1. Over 3 grams of fat (per 100 calories).

2. Over 800 milligrams of sodium.

3. Over 10 grams of refined sugar.

- Beware of the sugar and sodium in processed foods. Be sure to buy no/low sodium broths, soups, and canned veggies, and only buy canned fruit in its own juice.

- Throw away the seasoning packets in pasta, rice, and other boxed grain products and add your own favorite herbs and spices.

- Every packaged food item must have a nutrition facts panel. Be sure to read these labels for fat content. Keep the fat at 3 grams or less per 100 calories.

- Always use nonfat milk and light butter when preparing your boxed side dishes (i.e., scalloped potatoes, noodles, romanoff).

- Shop for your convenience foods at the local health or natural foods store. You'll find a variety of wholesome products with minimal preservatives.

- Venture over to your store's deli and/or butcher section to select prepared foods that aren't in a box.

Just make sure to choose items that are prepared with little fat.

▪ Scout out the restaurants in your area that offer healthy take-out meals. You can order ahead and pick it up on the way home from work.

DON'T GO TOO FAR WITH EATING IN THE CAR

The convenience of drive-thru restaurants fosters dining on the dash as well as the dashboard. This can be a blessing in your time-pressured world, but it's not a good habit to practice all of the time—mostly because it leaves you sitting too much. Then there are the crumbs and driblets to contend with.

Follow these tips and you can avoid any backlash of dining on the dash.

▪ Stock your car with a variety of healthy snacks (i.e., energy bars, a baggie of mixed cereal, carrot sticks, pretzels) that will make less of a mess.

▪ Keep at least two bottles of water with you in the car.

▪ Throw a few moisture wipes in your glove box for tidying up after your meal.

▪ When you're on a road trip, make sure you plan several stops for a little walk and stretch.

▪ Next time you're at a fast food restaurant, do your body a favor and skip the drive-thru. Park and go inside to place your order.

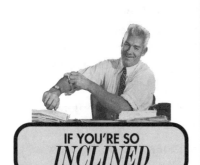

Be sure to incorporate the exercises described in Chapter 13, "Get Fit While You Sit," whenever you have to spend a lot of time in your car.

Congratulations! You're now roarin' down the road to healthiness, so give yourself a "brake" and plan the occasional detour with a stop at your favorite fast food joint for a low fat ice cream or shake.

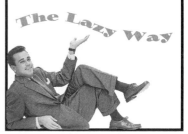

The Lazy Way

Getting Time on Your Side

	The Old Way	The Lazy Way
Looking at the menu	10 minutes	4 minutes
Ordering your meal	3 minutes	1 minute
Eating your meal	20 minutes	10 minutes (Half the time because you're eating half as much!)
Vending your way off the scale	Every day	Never again
Letting prepared foods box you out of your goals	Years	Not now, not ever!
Feeling guilty for that stop at McDonald's	Every time	No more!

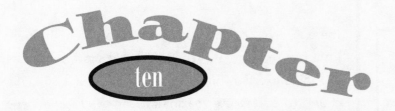

ten

Is Time on Your Side?

Tick-tock, tick-tock. Seconds slip into minutes . . . minutes move into hours . . . hours hurry into days. Each day that goes by seems to have less and less time. It's hard enough trying to find the time to get the "must do"s done, let alone sacrificing a single second on merely thinking about how to get the exercise in. Of course, that's the reason why weeks and months can pass before we get a chance to consider the "e" word. Well, the good news is it doesn't have to be a struggle at all. You just need to get a little time on your side.

This is easier to do than you think. First of all, banish the notion that you have to exercise three to five times a week, for 30 to 60 minutes, at around 60 percent to 90 percent of your maximum heart rate. Boy, you can get out of breath just trying to remember all of that! So, forget about it! Just let it go and leave it the masochists.

Instead, go for the easy-does-it alternative. Yes, you do need to get physical to shed some pounds, but 30 minutes a day is all it takes. And not even all at once. You can accumulate your activity throughout the day, a little here, a little

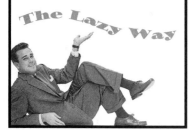

Congratulations! You've been up and "Adam" exercising five out of seven days this week. Be like Eve, a little sinful, and sleep in—you deserve it!

The Lazy Way

there. Exercise can be a snap when you break it up into little bits that fit your schedule. We'll show you how to slip some exertion time into your day. Be it a 10-minute chunk (the absolute maximum!) or a 30-second energizer during downtime, getting your exercise in has never been easier!

TAKE A BREATHER

When scheduling your exercise, nothing is more important than planning your day of rest. After all, if the Big Guy took a rest day, shouldn't we get one too? Of course! You deserve a day off (and if you're really busy, maybe an extra one).

But this needs to be planned. Look at your schedule for the week and decide which day is your busiest. That's the day you take a breather from exercising. Make sure you don't expend a smidgen of unnecessary energy on this day, and you shouldn't feel an ounce of guilt either!

BREAK THE BIG CHUNKS INTO LITTLE CHUNKS

You really can do a little here and a little there and still get the fringe benefits. You only need to break up that formidable "30-minute" chunk into little chunks that can work for you. Here are a few plans to ease exercise time into your schedule.

The Little Plan

The little plan consists of three 10-minute chunks. It works best for those of us who have a leisurely morning (this rules out anyone with children!), who can take a one-hour lunch and get home before the evening news. The first chunk fits in the morning before you have breakfast. The second chunk can be done at any time during your lunch break. The final chunk is completed as soon as you get home from work. The little plan may cause you to sweat a drop or two more, but it's worth it since you only have to find three slots in your schedule.

The Tiny Plan

The tiny plan is broken into six five-minute chunks. This design is good for those who have a tighter schedule but can fit in five minutes here and there. Do the first chunk as soon as you get up in the morning. The second chunk follows, during your mid-morning break. Get the third and fourth ones in at the top and bottom of your lunch hour. Number five fits in during your afternoon break, and the last chunk should be done after dinner.

The Teeny Plan

The teeny plan is made for those who are really pressed for time, and can only take a few minutes out of their schedule every now and then. It consists of 10 three-minute chunks. These tiny chunks fit in at the top of the hour, let's say from 8:00 in the morning to 5:00 in the evening. You can get your watch to beep on the hour to remind you. The beauty of the teeny plan is you don't have to deal with the beastly chore of changing a stitch of clothing because the teeny chunks of exertion tend to be pretty tame.

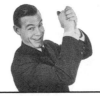

YOU'LL THANK YOURSELF LATER

It's as easy as one, two, three to gain muscle and lose fat more quickly! One: you can pick up your pace/intensity. Two: you can work out at the same speed for a longer duration. Three: you can add an extra workout per day or an extra exercise day per week.

DOWNTIME DOSES

We all have our downtime. Whether it's standing in the grocery line, waiting for the water to boil, or chatting on the phone, there are many moments in the day that provide us with a perfect opportunity to check out our fingernails or straighten our ties. We need this downtime. After all, when else can we perform such important tasks?

It's usually during these occasions that you notice the dirt specks on the floor or the scuffs on your shoes. Another thing you may note (besides how long it takes to send a fax) is the intense sleepiness that overcomes you, causing your mouth to gape and eyes to glaze over. These downtime moments can make you feel droopy, but if you add a touch of movement you can get energized and burn some calories at the same time.

Here are six effortless exercises that you can do in small doses so they'll fit right into your downtime.

The Un-Jumping Jack

This "jack" takes a lot less effort, and it's great for increasing the circulation in your upper body. It will loosen up your back and shoulders and invigorate you for your next task. Feel free to loosen your tie or take off your jacket when you do the unjumping jack (remember it's your downtime).

1. Stand with your feet shoulder-width apart, and the palms of your hands touching your thighs.

2. Raise arms up over your head, bringing palms together.

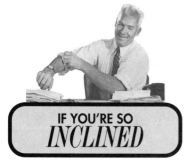

IF YOU'RE SO
INCLINED

Why stand still if you don't have to? Don't let someone else's schedule slow you down—use those idle moments to your advantage with simple exercises like the Un-Jumping Jack.

3. Bring arms back down to your thighs.

4. Repeat several times.

Un-jumping jacks are great for downtime in the copy room, at the fax machine, or during commercials.

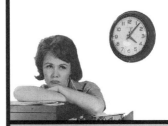

The Single Swinger

Swinging your legs is a great way to get the blood pumping in your lower extremities, and it's lots of fun. You may even find it's hard to stop yourself once you start the Single Swinger. Just make sure you balance it out and do it for both legs.

1. Stand next to a table or counter.

2. Turn to the right so your left hand is on the surface for support.

3. Keep hips even and tummy tucked, and begin swinging your right leg (keep it straight) first in front and then in back like a pendulum. Your supporting left leg should be slightly bent at the knee.

4. After 10 swings, turn and switch over to the other leg.

You can do the Single Swinger at your kitchen counter, while the microwave nukes your food, or even at the bathroom sink when you brush your teeth.

The Comfy Cat Stretch

You know how easy it is to build up tension in your neck, back, and shoulders, especially when you are working at your desk. Well, the Comfy Cat Stretch offers an easy way to get rid of it. You'll feel this stretch from your neck to your arm sockets.

1. Stand behind a sturdy chair or desk.

2. Place both paws on the surface, shoulder-width apart.

3. Step back, bending at the waist, and drop your head forward, keeping your chin close to your chest.

4. Push your rear back as if someone was pulling your tail.

The Comfy Cat Stretch is a purrfect one for downtime while your document prints or the credit card company has you hanging on hold.

The Stationary Jogger

This little exercise is great for when you're all dressed up with no where to go! That's because you basically stay in one place. The Stationary Jogger gets you moving without you having to take a single step forward, backward or sideways.

1. Stand up straight as if being pulled up by a string.

2. Bend the right knee, rolling the weight of your leg to the ball of your foot, bringing your right heel up.

3. Now roll back down on your heel, bending your left knee at the same time.

4. Alternate legs rolling back in forth from toe to heel.

5. You can burn a couple extra calories by using your arms too. Swing the opposite arm with opposite leg.

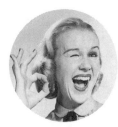

QUICK **n** PAINLESS

Stuck at the curb? Try the Stationary Jogger and keep your blood moving, even if you're not!

Use the Stationary Jogger for lulls behind shopping carts or in front of ATMs.

The Two-Legged Flamingo

You might not look as graceful as a flamingo when doing this exercise, but we're pretty sure you would prefer your legs over a bird's. Anyway, you don't need grace to perform this simple feat, and it's a great way to firm the calves.

1. Keeping your body straight, raise both heels from the floor until you are standing on your toes. Use a desk or wall for support if balance becomes a problem.

2. Lower slowly and repeat 10 times.

3. If you want to be a one-legged flamingo (more advanced), do one leg at a time by wrapping your other foot around the ankle to be raised.

You can do the Two-Legged Flamingo whenever you're standing around, whether you're in the water or on dry land.

The Royal Rope Climber

The Royal Rope Climber is another great stretch to help ease the tension in your body. One of the best times to do this stretch is when you first wake up in the morning (after your longest downtime). A word of warning though: It may cause you to yawn more than usual.

1. You can do this stretch standing or sitting, but lying down is best.

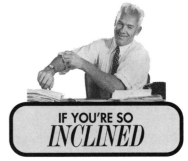

IF YOU'RE SO
INCLINED

Looking for a little more? Try the One-Legged Flamingo to push yourself a bit harder!

2. Pretend you have a rope dangling right in front of you. If you are lying down, the rope is above and behind you.

3. Reach up with one hand as high as you can on the imaginary rope.

4. Then pull this rope down to your side.

5. Now reach up with your other hand and pull it down.

6. As you alternate your hands you will feel a soothing stretch in your sides.

You'll love doing the Royal Rope Climber in bed, but it is also a good one for downtime at the little league game. In fact, you can add a few whoops and you'll be cheering *The Lazy Way*.

WORKING OUT IN A WINK

Why is it that so many people will get in their cars and drive to the local health club just so they can get on a treadmill to walk for one mile? Seems like twice the work with half the return.

You carry your legs with you wherever you go, so why not wear your favorite sneakers and go for a stroll when you feel like it? No car keys. No gym clothes. No membership card. Just you and your sneakers. Getting the exercises in wherever you happen to be can save you a lot of time, energy, and gas too! That's why we gear all of the activities described in the following chapters to be done on the spot, whatever and whenever you fancy.

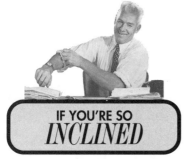

IF YOU'RE SO
INCLINED

Pooped after the first block? Add a little pep to your pace. Use books on tape to exercise your mind while you work on your body. The minutes will slip by as the fat slides off.

Another way you can shave off several minutes is by combining movements when toning your muscles. You won't have to worry about traffic jams or fancy equipment or overdoing it either. There's no need to give each muscle its own set of reps. They are perfectly content with being addressed and stimulated as a group (it's their bonding time, so to speak). So you can get right to pushing and pulling with only half of the panting. If you want to get back to work in a blink, don't forget the tips we gave you on tidying up after your workout (see Chapter 5). They'll help you save time and probably lots of water.

Working out *The Lazy Way* is all about getting time on your side. It's breaking the big chunks into smaller chunks that you can handle. It's taking advantage of your downtime. It's using what you've got on the spot. Combine all of these elements and you'll drift painlessly through your workout.

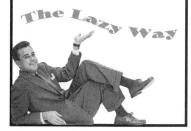

Congratulations! You've been using what you've got on the spot! Now find your favorite spot and enjoy a little quiet time—you deserve it!

Getting Time on Your Side

	The Old Way	The Lazy Way
Fitting exercise time in	30 to 60 minutes	3 to 10 minutes
Toning your muscles	30 to 45 minutes	10 to 15 minutes
Getting ready for your workout	5 to 8 minutes	1 minute, tops!
Getting going in the morning	Impossible!	5 minutes
Keeping going in the afternoon	It can't be done!	5 minutes
Being idle when stuck in the aisle	All the time	Never again!

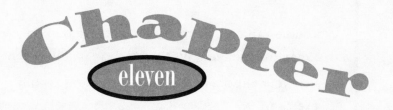

eleven

Molding Your Muscles in Minutes

Your muscles are your best friends when it comes to shedding pounds. And the more you have, the easier and more permanent your pound shedding will be. You want to keep these friends around for life. After all, they support you, keep you balanced, and give you strength to lose weight. They are not even high maintenance . . . all they ask of you is a little nourishment, lots of stimulation, and some time to rest.

So, how can you gather these sinewy friends around you without feeling too bound or bulged out? It doesn't take much—just a few props and a few minutes. But, there are also a few guidelines you should follow to get the maximum benefit from your muscles. Here are some things to remember as you begin molding your muscles:

- You only need to strength train two to three times per week.

- Do one to two sets of 12 to 15 repetitions.

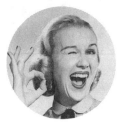

- Your last three repetitions should be hard to do. When they get easy, it's time to increase the weight.

- Rest your muscles at least 48 hours after strength exercises.

- Use proper breathing. Blow out during the hard part of the exercise, and breathe in during the easy part.

- Always keep your abdominal muscles pulled in and stabilize your body with all exercises.

- Stretch slowly and gradually, up to a point of tension—never bounce!

- Hold your stretches for a count of 30 to 50.

- Never strength train or stretch your muscles without warming up first (i.e., do 5 to 10 minutes of easy walking before or after your aerobic workout).

Now, here's something you can forget about . . . going to the gym! (That is unless you want to.) You can mold your muscles in the comfort of your own home with a few dumbbells and/or some elastic tubing and a couple of pieces of furniture (see Chapter 2 for more details). Then, there's the most important piece of equipment—your body!

YOUR OWN BOD IS THE BEST TOOL TO PROD

The greatest machine to mold your muscles *The Lazy Way* is your very own body. It's cheap, convenient, long-lasting, and hopefully it's not too squeaky or in need of repair. But, there's another fine reason why you should not resist using your body as a resistance tool. When you rely on your own body for strength training, you force it to stabilize itself rather than a machine stabilizing it. This will improve your balance and coordination.

Using your body for resistance also allows you to work several muscle groups at the same time. For instance, if you used a leg extension machine, you would be targeting your quadriceps (front of thighs), but if you used your body to do a "kneel down," you would target your quadriceps, hamstrings (back of thighs), and buttocks muscles. So, take advantage of this incredible machine you carry around with you. Follow the exercises in this chapter, and you'll see it doesn't take much to prod your bod.

MUSCLE TONING WITHOUT THE GROANING

There's no need to groan about the following strength exercises. They're simple, quick, and very effective. So, get ready to mold your muscles from head to toe. (Note: Do the exercises in the order we give them; that way you'll work your bigger muscle groups first.)

Moves for Your Upper Body

The following exercises will strengthen and tone your back, chest, shoulders, and arms.

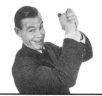

YOU'LL THANK YOURSELF LATER

It keeps going and going and going. Just like that little Energizer bunny, a smidgen more exercise can go a long way toward a healthier you. Muscle cells burn calories and produce energy, and they continue to burn calories well after you stop exercising.

Sitting Down Pulls

1. Sit on the floor with your legs out in front of you, keeping your back straight and abdominals pulled in.

2. Wrap elastic tubing around your feet and hold the ends of the tubing in each hand, with your arms extended in front of you.

3. With your knees slightly bent, slowly pull your arms toward your waist, pushing your chest out and squeezing your shoulder blades together. Keep your abdominals tight so that your lower back doesn't arch.

4. Slowly return to the starting position and repeat for the desired number of times.

5. You can make this exercise harder by shortening the length of elastic tubing (wrap more of it around your hand).

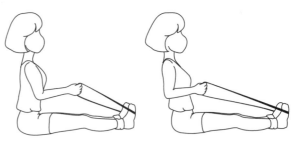

Figure 12.1: Sitting Down Pulls: Try this one next time you're sitting in front of the TV!

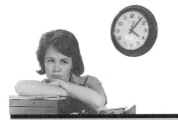

Lounging Lizard Lifts

These lifts can be done at three levels (from easy to difficult).

Level 1: Off the Wall

1. Stand about an arm's length away from a wall, palms against the wall about chest height, knees slightly bent.

2. Keeping your neck, head, and back straight and your abdominals tight, slowly bend your elbows and lean forward until your forehead touches the wall.

3. Pause for a second, then use your arm and shoulder muscles to push back to the starting position.

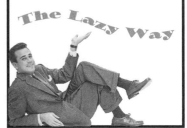

Congratulations! You've mastered the Lounging Lizard Lift! Take a break and enjoy some nice lemonade!

The Lazy Way

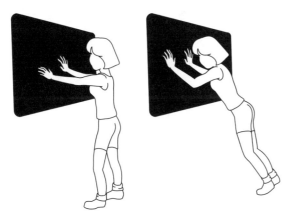

Figure 12.2A: Lounging Lizard Lifts: Start with the easy version first!

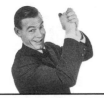

Use it or lose it! Women (and men) need to build strength in their shoulders and chest to keep their upper bodies from sagging over time. Your best move would be to incorporate push-ups three days a week into your workout or go the totally *Lazy Way* and just buy a Wonder Bra (it may be difficult to find in men's sizes).

Level 2: On Your Knees

1. Kneel on all fours on a padded floor, hands about shoulder-width apart and positioned slightly forward of your shoulders, feet facing back with toes flat on the floor.

2. Press your hips down to keep your torso in a straight line and keep your abdominals pulled in.

3. Slowly bend your elbows and lower your body as a unit, chest and chin moving down to nearly touch the floor. Then push back up. Don't lock your elbows.

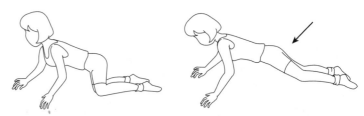

Figure 12.2B: Lounging Lizard Lifts Too: Ready for a little more? This version is a little tougher!

Level 3: On Your Toes

1. On a padded floor, balance your weight on your hands and feet. Hands are about shoulder-width apart and positioned slightly forward of your shoulders. Your legs are extended straight back, supported by the balls of your feet. Keep your torso in a straight line.

2. Slowly and smoothly bend your elbows and lower body as a unit, chest and chin moving down to nearly touch the floor.

3. Then push back up. Don't lock your elbows.

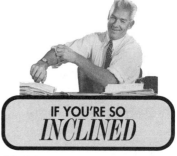

IF YOU'RE SO
INCLINED

Making the grade. Keep track of how many repetitions you can do of one set of exercises for each half of your body (upper and lower). As you progress, give yourself a pop quiz and see if you've made the grade (surpassed your original number). It may be time to graduate to the next level!

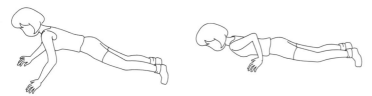

Figure 12.2C: More Lounging Lizard Lifts: Okay, you're ready for it! It's time for Advanced Lizard!

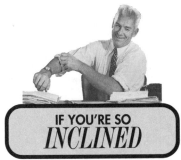

You don't need any special equipment to create your own thigh buster. Grab your own homemade dumbbells and do some walking lunges to the mailbox and back.

Lying Down Arm Raises

1. Lie on your side with your legs straight and your top arm stretched out in front of you.

2. Hold a light weight with your top hand and slowly raise your straight arm toward the ceiling. Do not go beyond your body's midline.

3. Slowly bring your arm back down.

4. Repeat for the desired number of repetitions, then turn onto your other side and lift your other arm.

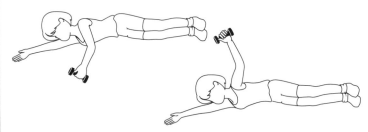

Figure 12.3: Lying Down Arm Raises: Who says you can't lie down on the job? Sprawl out in your favorite room and give this a try!

Moves for Your Lower Body

The following exercises will strengthen and tone your buttocks, thighs, and lower legs.

Sit Downs

1. Stand erect in front of your kitchen counter with feet about shoulder-width apart, toes pointing straight forward, hands gripping the counter for balance.

2. Keep your back straight and your heels flat on the floor.

3. Slowly bend your knees, up to a 90-degree angle (thighs will be horizontal), while pressing down on your little toes and keeping your knees over the feet as much as possible.

4. Then straighten to original position.

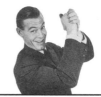

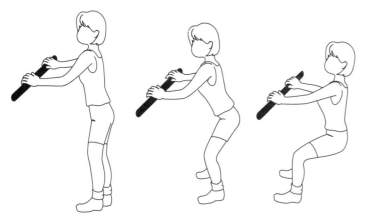

Figure 12.4: Sit Downs: Got a few minutes of standing around? Break up the monotony with this one!

YOU'LL THANK YOURSELF LATER

Diversify your workout and your fun. Keeping your exercise exciting is half the battle (the other half is getting into your lycra shorts). Remember to vary the type of exercise you do from day to day, and as you get more fit (and want to venture outside), add new types of workouts to your exercise routine.

Kneel Downs

1. Stand with feet slightly apart, toes forward, knees relaxed, and arms down at your sides.

2. Move one foot forward with back leg balancing on the ball of back foot. Your back heel should be off the floor, and your back knee should be slightly bent. This is your starting position.

3. Next, start lowering your body to the floor by bending your front knee. It's important to come down as if you are balancing a jug of water on your head (shoulders over hips, front knee aligned with front foot). Keep your arms at your sides.

4. Return to the starting position and repeat for the desired number of repetitions.

5. Then change legs and repeat this exercise.

6. Advanced version: hold dumbbells at your sides.

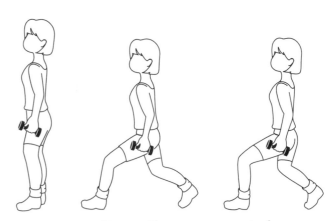

Figure 12.5: Kneel Downs: This is a great exercise for thighs, calves, and abs!

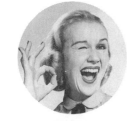

QUICK 🔘 PAINLESS

Stuck in line? Try the Kneel Down exercise while you're waiting and keep your blood pumping!

Lying Down Arches

1. Lie on your back with your arms straight out at your sides, with both knees bent and both feet flat on the floor.

2. Keeping your upper back on the floor, slowly raise your buttocks until there is an imaginary straight line from your shoulders to your knees.

3. Then slowly lower your pelvis back to the floor. Don't arch your back.

4. Repeat this for the desired number of repetitions.

5. For a variation on this exercise, place a ball between your knees and squeeze the ball as you come up and down. This works your inner thighs.

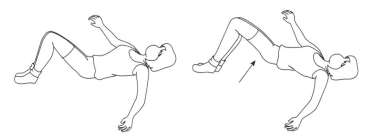

Figure 12.6: Lying Down Arches: This one is great for abs, thighs, calves, and buns . . . Who knew it could be this easy?

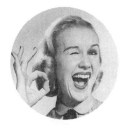

QUICK ⬭ PAINLESS

Squeeze me, please. If you were an abdominal muscle and you felt some exercise coming on what would be your first reaction?

1. Trying to find yourself.

2. Just hanging out.

3. Uptight and out of sight.

For your sake (and your body's) we hope you chose #3.

Don't Forget Your Middle!

Your abdominals are probably your most important muscular friends. They help your posture, protect your vital organs, stabilize your torso, and support your lower back. So you definitely want to have strong abdominals! Here are some easy moves for your middle.

Pull Ins

1. Lie on your back with your knees bent and your feet flat on the floor (alternately, you can have your legs on a chair and your knees at right angles).

2. Inhale deeply, allowing your middle to expand.

3. Now, slowly exhale and at the same time tilt your hips upward, pressing you back down onto the floor. Don't let your hips come off the floor.

4. Contract your abdomen (pulling your belly button closer to your spine) while exhaling. It's important to keep your belly flat and force all the air out because this is what works the deepest layers of your abs.

5. Then relax and breathe in. Repeat.

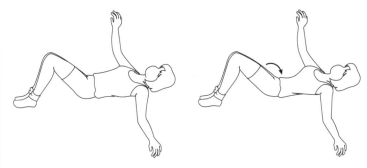

Figure 12.7: Pull Ins: Time to get deep into those abs!

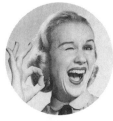

QUICK ⬭ PAINLESS

Take a stand (or a seat) on your middle ground. Crunches can increase or decrease your middle. Crunching on food will increase your middle, but doing crunches on the floor during commercial breaks, on the lawn when you're outside playing with the kids, or in the car as you're waiting for traffic to unsnarl can decrease your middle.

Slide Ups

1. Lie on your back with your knees bent and your feet about shoulder-width apart.

2. Cup your left hand under your head. Place your right hand across and onto the outer part of your left thigh.

3. Keeping both hips on the ground, contract your abdomen and slide your right hand upward along your left thigh.

4. Hold this for a count of five.

5. Exhale as you contract and raise your hand, inhale as you come down and relax.

6. Repeat the mirror image of this, placing your left hand on your right thigh.

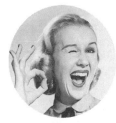

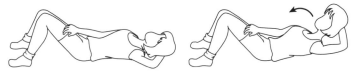

Figure 12.8: Slide Ups: Since you're already on the floor, move onto this one and continue to work those abs!

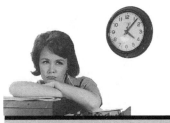

MUSCLE STRETCHING WITHOUT THE WRETCHING

You can stretch your muscles without much strain. All you have to do is relax! The following moves will soothe tired muscles and improve poor posture.

Moves for Your Upper Body

The following stretches will loosen and relax your neck and upper torso.

Neck Unleashers

1. Stand erect, with your arms dangling at your sides.

2. Tilt your head to your right side. Lower your right ear to your right shoulder while keeping your shoulders down. Hold this position.

3. Then repeat to the left side.

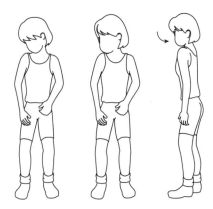

Figure 12.9: Neck Unleashers: This one you can do anywhere you have to stand up . . . at the grocery store, doing the dishes, waiting for the bathroom in the morning . . .

4. Turn your head to the right with chin pointing toward shoulders (shoulders remain still). Hold this position.

5. Repeat this to the left side.

6. Pull in your chin to make a "double" chin, stretching the back of your neck. Hold this position. CAUTION: Do not lift your chin up and tilt your head back while doing this—it hyperextends your neck.

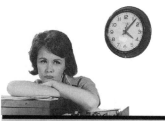

Shoulder Slackeners

1. Move your shoulders in a circle.

2. Start with five forward circles, then five backward circles.

3. Stretch your right arm across your chest with your left hand pressing against your right shoulder. Hold this position.

4. Repeat with left arm.

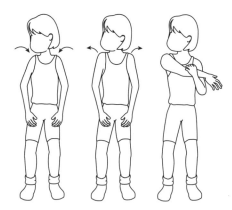

Figure 12.10: Shoulder Slackeners: Still stuck in line somewhere? Do this for five minutes and kill some time!

Upper Back Unbinders

1. Bending your elbows, interlock your fingers in front of your chest, palms outward.

2. Push your arms forward, straightening your arms and rounding your upper back. Hold this position. Then release it.

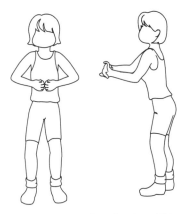

Figure 12.11: Upper Back Unbinders: This one is so easy, it doesn't even feel like exercise!

Moves for Your Lower Body

The following stretches will loosen and relax your lower back, hips, and legs.

Knee Huggers

1. Lie on your back with your knees bent, feet flat on the floor, and your arms straight out to the sides.

2. Bring your knees toward your chest and keep them bent at a right angle, hugging them with your arms. Hold this position.

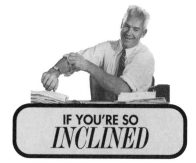

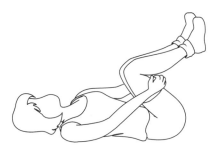

Figure 12.12: Knee Huggers: This is a great one for everyone who gets stuck sitting all day . . . stretch out that lower back!

IF YOU'RE SO

INCLINED

Long day at the office? Try the Knee Hugger and stretch out your back!

Plop Overs

1. Start with the Knee Huggers, but leave your arms straight out to the sides.

2. Keeping both shoulders on the floor, slowly let your legs fall to the right side until your right leg is resting on the floor. Hold this position.

3. Repeat on the other side.

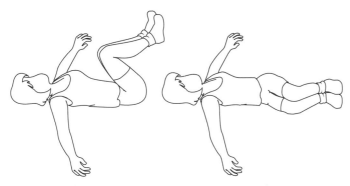

Figure 12.13: Plop Overs: No, it's not a breakfast item, just another great way to work on those lower back muscles!

Hip Unflexors

1. Get down on your left knee as if you were going to propose marriage. Your right knee should be at a right angle to the floor, with the knee over the ankle.

2. Without moving your right leg, press your hips forward until you feel a stretch in the upper part of your left thigh. Don't let your back arch.

3. Repeat with the other leg.

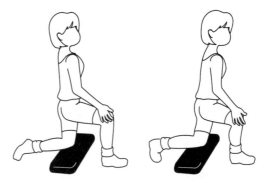

Figure 12.14: Hip Unflexors: This is another great, low-impact exercise for the lower back and hip area.

Ease Into Its

1. Stand erect, with your arms dangling at your sides.

2. Step forward on your left foot, with your right leg resting on toes pointed straight forward.

3. Press your right heel to the floor, keeping your left knee aligned over your left ankle. To deepen the stretch, slide your right foot farther backward. Hold this position.

4. Now, slightly bend your back knee without lifting your heel. Hold this position.

5. Repeat the same process for the other side.

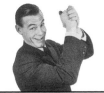

Just because you're still waiting doesn't mean you have to be still! Work these exercises into your idle moments and make the most of it!

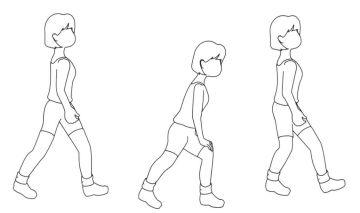

Figure 12.15: Ease Into Its: Waiting for your kids to get out of school? Do this one while you wait, and keep those muscles working, even when you have to stay in one place!

Don't Forget Your Middle!

Your middle and lower back can get really tight, especially if you have to sit all day. These stretches will help lengthen your spine and relieve any stress on your back.

Up and Down Arches

1. Get on your hands and knees.

2. First arch your back up like a scared cat. Pull your stomach in and hold this position.

3. Then lower your back until it bows in the middle. Hold this position.

4. Repeat as many times as you like.

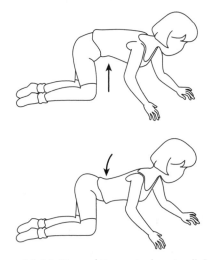

Figure 12.16: Up and Down Arches: Is all that sitting at the office making you think you're getting shorter? Stretch that spine out with this one!

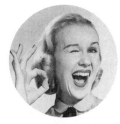

QUICK 🔘 PAINLESS

A few seconds here and there will help you and your back make it through another day. Be good to yourself!

Back Releasers

1. Lie on your stomach with your palms on the floor slightly forward of your shoulders.

2. Relax your back, and slowly press up your body for a good back and abdominal stretch.

3. Keep hips on floor and eyes looking straight ahead (not up). Hold this position.

4. Then lower yourself. In the event of lower back pain, either do not lift as high or discontinue the stretch.

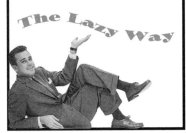

Congratulations! You've learned some easy exercises to get fit, now exercise your brain and read a good book!

The Lazy Way

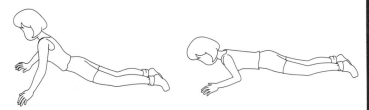

Figure 12.17: Back Releasers: Almost as good as a massage, this exercise will make a difference when it comes to a stressed-out back!

Getting Time on Your Side

	The Old Way	The Lazy Way
Your muscle molding routine	30 to 45 minutes	10 to 15 minutes
Your stretching routine	10 to 15 minutes	5 to 8 minutes
Your ab crunching routine	10 minutes	4 minutes
Getting to the gym to work out	30 minutes	Never again!
Finding the equipment you need to work out	Weeks	Don't need any!
Feeling a difference	Months	Half the time!

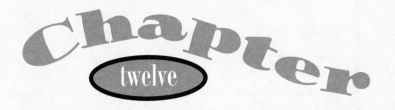

Stir Up the Calories

There's no doubt about it . . . if you want to shed some pounds, you definitely need to rouse those calories into motion. But the good news is you don't have to whip your-self into a frenzy to get results. You don't even have to churn those calories all at once. Rather, you can smolder them one at a time whenever you like.

It's okay to choose an activity that won't excite your body too much, but it's crucial to pick something you enjoy doing. Keeping active is the key to permanent weight loss, so your activity needs to be enjoyable, convenient, and endurable. In this chapter, we'll give you the tips and tools you'll need to make your exercise work without leaving you feeling too worked.

MELTING THE FAT WITHOUT BURNING YOURSELF OUT

There are a few things you'll want to know before you start stirring up the calories. What type of activity is best along with just how much and how hard you have to do it are some of the tips we're going to give you. But first, we want to go over some fat-burning principles.

Simmering Down Some Fat-Burning Facts

When we talk about exercising to burn fat, we use the term aerobic, which means in the presence of oxygen. You cannot burn fat without oxygen. When you do aerobic exercise, you increase your aerobic capacity or your ability to take in, transport, and utilize oxygen. Increasing your aerobic capacity helps you become a better fat burner.

Here are some guidelines to remember when you exercise aerobically:

- Choose an activity that is continuous and uses your larger muscle groups. Examples of these activities are dancing, walking, jogging, biking, and swimming.

- Pick at least two or three activities and rotate them. Variety will keep you from getting bored or injured.

- Begin slowly and gradually progress in effort, frequency, and duration (no more than 10 percent increase per week).

- Wear the right kind of shoes and clothing.

- Always warm up before and cool down after your aerobic exercise (easy pace for at least five minutes).

Little Chunks, Tiny Chunks, Teeny Chunks

We've told you that you don't need to do more than 30 minutes, five to six days a week. And, you don't have to

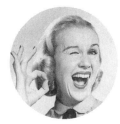

QUICK n° PAINLESS

Doing the time warp. Don't forget that walking for 10 minutes three times a day can burn the same amount of calories as one 30-minute walk. Keep the seconds on your side and don't get caught in a time warp.

exercise all at once. You can break it up into little chunks, tiny chunks, or teeny chunks (see Chapter 11). You will see results if you do this, especially if you haven't been doing anything up to this point.

Of course, you see even more results if you increase those chunks of time. The more you exercise, the more calories and fat you burn—even after you stop. The choice is yours to make, but if you decide to stick with the smaller chunks of time, be sure to use as many muscle groups as you can. For instance, pick whole body activities like rowing, cross country skiing, jumping rope, or jumping jacks. Remember, the more muscles you use, the less time you need to move them.

With a Huff and a Puff You'll Blow That Fat Down

In order to get the benefits of aerobic exercise, you need to get your heart beating at a level beyond its resting state and below its maximum rate. That means you will get a little heated, a little breathless, and a little sweaty (or really sweaty depending on your plumbing). Sounds like fun, huh?!

Seriously though, you need to listen to your body and work at a level of exertion that feels moderate to hard. On a scale from 1 to 10, this exertion level will be at $7\frac{1}{2}$ to $8\frac{1}{2}$. Remember that how you feel exercising today may be different from tomorrow, so always pay attention to your breathing and energy level. If you want an actual target zone for working out turn to the table at the end of this chapter to calculate these numbers.

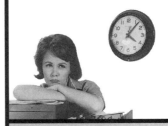

A COMPLETE WASTE OF TIME

The 3 Worst Ways to Kill Your Energy/ Excitement Level:

1. Work out too vigorously in the beginning (start small and build).

2. Do the same activity over and over (vary your workout routine).

3. Injure yourself (purchase the appropriate footwear/gear for your activities).

It's a complete waste of time to start off with a bang and end with a whimper.

Stirring Up a Melting Pot of Benefits

Exercise does a lot more for you then melting fat and calories. It truly is the cornerstone of good health and a productive life. There are so many benefits for working out (even if you do it *The Lazy Way*). Once you see them you'll probably never want to stop stirring those calories.

Here are a dozen ways aerobic exercise improves your life:

- Decreases stress
- Lowers blood pressure
- Stabilizes blood sugar
- Reduces unhealthy blood fats and increases healthy ones
- Raises HDL cholesterol levels
- Increases endurance
- Enhances balance and coordination
- Decreases appetite
- Improves resistance to disease
- Makes bones stronger
- Aids restful, higher-quality sleep
- Helps slow the aging process

And, don't forget, when it comes to shedding pounds, the more you increase your aerobic capacity, the better fat burner you become.

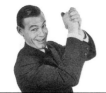

YOU'LL THANK YOURSELF LATER

The beat goes on . . . To check if you're at your training level count your pulse beats at your neck or wrist for 15 seconds. Multiply the number of beats by four. That's your beats per minute.

Your Aerobic Activity Can Be a Walk in the Park

You know we carry our legs with us wherever we go, so we might as well make the most of them. One of the best ways to do this is to make walking the aerobic activity of choice. There are a multitude of ways you can fit walking into your routine. It just takes some imagination and a good pair of tennies.

Here's how you can cultivate the pleasures of walking.

- Find a rewarding place to walk. It can be your neighborhood, a green belt, a beach, or the nearest park (if it's a small one, walk around the perimeter).

- Take a walk first thing in the morning and see a part of the day you might usually miss.

- Go for a walk in the great outdoors during your lunch break. It will feel good to breathe in some fresh air.

- Change some of your regular driving routes into walking ones. Take your legs instead of your car to work, school, or to visit a friend or buy a newspaper.

- Head for the shopping malls and walk from end to end! (Sorry, but window shopping doesn't count!) The shopping malls are a great place to walk when the weather is bad.

- Get yourself a portable headset so that you can listen to music or books on tape.

- Walk with a friend. (Don't forget dogs enjoy walks, too!)

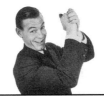

YOU'LL THANK YOURSELF LATER

Now you see it, now you don't! Consider it your own brand of 'slight of hand.' You can have that double scoop of Rocky Road ice cream you're craving as long as you acknowledge the time and energy it will cost to make it disappear. You may decide it doesn't look so magical after all.

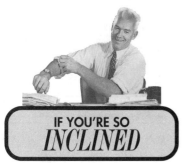

Frank did it "his way" but you can do it your way. Venture off the beaten path. Hike up hills, climb down rugged terrain, or walk on sand to increase your workout without adding time.

A SPURT HERE AND THERE DOES WONDERS FOR MORE THAN JUST YOUR DERRIÈRE

We told you that there was no need to whip yourself into a frenzy and we meant it. But, we should also tell you that adding a spurt of effort every now and then while exercising can do wonders for your pound shedding. These spurts are an efficient way to get your body fit and rev up your fat-burning potential. And, because it's just a spurt, you don't have time to get bent out of shape.

It's easy to incorporate these spurts into your exercise routine. After you've been doing your activity for several minutes, increase your intensity for 30 to 60 seconds, then bring it back down to your normal pace. For instance, if you are walking, you might walk faster or break into a jog for a little bit. This can be applied to whatever activity you choose—just do it a little harder or faster and let yourself get uncomfortable, and then return to your regular pace, breathing comfortably before starting another spurt.

Here are a few ideas to help you rev it up every now and then:

- Find a hill or overpass
- Do 20 step-ups on a bench (10 on each leg)
- Run up a flight of stairs
- Do stride outs between telephone poles
- Skip, leap, or bound

- Increase the intensity or resistance on cardiovascular machines
- Add hand weights to your work out

JUST A LITTLE MORE MOVEMENT YIELDS A LOT MORE RESULTS

A spurt of intensity will definitely increase your calorie expenditure, but just a little more movement yields results too, especially nowadays, since technology has made our lives more efficient but less active. You need to figure out how you can be more active during the day, from the time you wake up until the time you go to bed. Try to add a little physical activity everywhere you go.

Here are some simple ways to get more physical:

- Never choose the closest parking space—walk a bit to where you're going.
- Always take the stairs over the elevator or escalator.
- Promise yourself you'll pull five weeds a day from your yard.
- Plant a garden or flowers.
- Use your manual can opener rather than the electric one.
- Learn to fidget while you sit (see the next chapter for more details).
- Never sit during commercial breaks. Get up and move around.
- Incorporate down time exercises whenever you can.

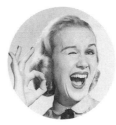

QUICK ☜ⁿ☞ PAINLESS

Move over soul train, here comes the interval train. It's got rhythm, soul, and a whole lot more. To incorporate interval training into your workout, add short bursts of high intensity exercise to your regular routine. For example, walk three minutes at your regular pace and then speed up for one minute. You can adjust your rhythm and intensity as your exercise tolerance increases.

A TREAT FOR A FEAT

There are going to be times when you will indulge your-self with a decadent treat, especially during the holidays or on special occasions. It's quite okay to do this every now and then, after all, you should never deprive your-self. But, there's a way to make it seem like you never ate those extra calories. Just exchange your treat for a feat!

Amount of Minutes for Different Body Weights

Treat (calories)	Feat	**Pounds**				
		120	**140**	**160**	**180**	**200**
Alcoholic beverage (110)	Walking (brisk)	24	19	17	15	14
2" square brownie (96)	Biking	26	23	20	17	16
1 oz. candy bar (130)	Tennis (singles)	24	21	18	16	14
1 slice cheesecake (200)	Skating	30	26	23	20	18
1 oz. chips (150)	Dancing (aerobic)	18	15	13	12	11
Croissant (167)	Rowing	24	20	18	16	14
Donut (cake type) (55)	Ping-Pong	16	14	12	11	9
French fries (small) (270)	Jogging	30	26	23	20	18
4 oz. ice cream (135)	Basketball	18	17	15	13	12
Nachos (regular) (346)	Jumping rope	48	41	36	32	29
1 oz. nuts (159)	Swimming	22	19	16	14	13
1 slice of pie (173)	Hiking	32	28	25	22	20

SHED SOME POUNDS The Lazy Way

As you can see, it takes quite a feat to get rid of your treat. The good news is you don't have to complete the minutes all at once. You can divide the time up in chunks just like your exercise routine. Feel free to make a copy of this table and post it in a useful place—the refrigerator or pantry door for example.

The preceding table shows the amount of calories for various treats along with the number of minutes it would take to burn them off. The table assumes that you would perform each activity at the perceived exertion level of moderate to hard.

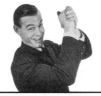

YOU'LL THANK YOURSELF LATER

Put this table on your fridge, or even in your snack drawer at work, so you can keep track!

Getting Time on Your Side

	The Old Way	The Lazy Way
Your aerobic routine	30 to 60 minutes	10 minutes max
Your high-intensity training	2 to 5 minutes	30 to 60 seconds
Pulling weeds in your yard	Half a day	5 minutes
Working your biceps	30 minutes at the gym	10 minutes in the kitchen (putting groceries away)
Getting in a run	30 minutes at the gym	15 minutes at home chasing your toddler
Working your upper body	40 minutes at the gym	15 minutes at home washing the windows

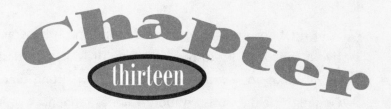

Chapter
thirteen

Get Fit While You Sit

Sitting is the most popular posture in our society. So popular, that some of us will even stand in line and wait to be seated. With today's technology, there's no need to run all around. You can do almost anything from your computer, car, or couch. Heck, you can even get fit while you sit!

It would be a bummer if you didn't take advantage of all the time you spend on your seat to burn more calories. After all, wouldn't you rather burn your calories sitting down instead of running around? We'll show you an effortless way to ward off the spread and give you some simple exercises you can do right from your chair.

YOU'LL HAVE LESS TO FEAR IF YOU FIDGET ON YOUR REAR

Even though sitting is easy, it's hard on your body. Sitting puts a lot of stress on your back and hinders your posture and circulation. That's why it's important to get up and move around every half hour or so to relieve your muscles and joints and get your blood flowing. But, there's something you can do to help yourself if you need to sit for a long time—just fidget!

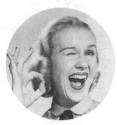

Fidgeting is not only for when someone is hyperactive or needs to go to the bathroom. It is an effortless activity that you can incorporate into your sitting time. Fidgeting helps you burn more calories, enhances your circulation, and lightens the stress load on your back. So promise yourself to fidget every chance you get.

Here are some classic fidgeting moves to help you get started:

Thigh Flaps

Keeping your feet flat on the floor and your abdominals pulled in, flap your thighs toward the center and then outward. Repeat continuously.

Jitter Bugs

Come up on the balls of your feet and move your legs as if you are shivering or trembling. Place your palms on your thighs and start rolling your shoulders back as you continue to move your legs.

Toe Taps

Keeping your feet flat on the floor and your abdominals pulled in, flex your right foot so that it rests on your right heel then bring it down tapping your foot on the floor. Now do your left foot. Alternate movement from side to side.

Roly-Polys

Move from side to side on your chair, raising your hip up toward the ceiling. Repeat continuously.

A DOZEN MOVES YOU CAN DO FROM YOUR CHAIR

We have some great news for those of you who seem to be stuck in your chairs. There's no reason why you can't strengthen and tone your whole body from your bottom (on up). Most of the exercises can be done using your own body as resistance. A couple of dumbbells (home-made or store-bought), ankle weights, and elastic tubing are great tools to add to your seated workout.

Here are a dozen simple exercises that will make you feel cheeky in no time:

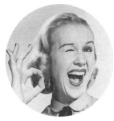

QUICK ━━ PAINLESS

Doing the hokey pokey. You put your right foot in, you put your right foot out, you put your right foot in and you move it all about. That's what its all about. Things haven't changed much since kindergarten. Move it and you'll lose it.

Bottom Ups

1. Position yourself in your chair so that your feet are firmly planted on the floor (you may need to move forward a little). Feet should be shoulder-width apart.

2. Without moving your torso forward too much, go from a seated position to a standing one.

3. Come back down into a seated position. Repeat 10 to 15 times.

   Note: You may need to use your arms to help you at first. As your legs get stronger try not to use your arms at all.

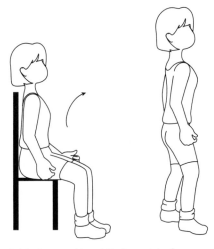

Figure 14.1: Bottom Ups: Hit that mid-afternoon lull? Try this one! It'll get you going for the home stretch!

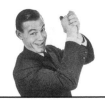

Pedal Pushers

1. Lean back and scoot your fanny forward so that it rests at the edge of your chair. Be sure to keep your abdominals pulled in.

2. Extend your legs in front of you and start pedaling them as if you were riding a bicycle.

3. Don't forget to breathe and keep your abdominals pulled in tightly.

4. Pedal for 20 to 30 cycles.

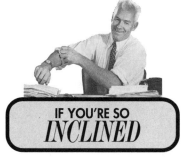

IF YOU'RE SO
INCLINED

Try the exercises from this chapter when you first get into work and you'll be starting off on the right foot!

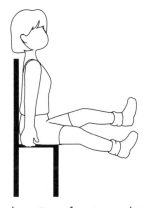

Figure 14.2: Pedal Pushers: Even if you're stuck in traffic, at least these exercises will help you feel as if you are getting somewhere!

Cross Overs

1. Lean back and scoot your fanny forward so that it rests at the edge of your chair. Be sure to keep your abdominals pulled in.

2. Extend your legs straight in front of you.

3. Begin Cross Overs by moving your straight legs outward as wide as possible.

4. Bring your legs back in, crossing over each other in the middle.

5. Then move legs outward again, this time crossing under each other when they come back to the middle.

6. Alternate crossing legs over and under each other 15 to 20 times.

7. Don't forget to breathe and to keep your abdominals pulled in tightly.

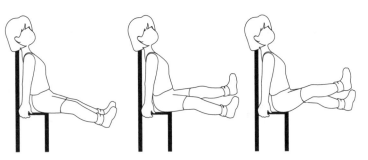

Figure 14.3: Cross Overs: Stuck in a long conference call? Try these exercises . . . go ahead! No one can see you anyway!

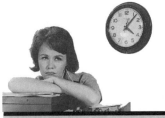

A COMPLETE WASTE OF TIME

The 3 Worst Ways to Achieve Proper Posture Are:

1. Keep your abdominals loose.

2. Keep your back curved (slouched).

3. Keep your legs crossed.

Squeezers

1. Sit up straight with abdominals pulled in and feet planted firmly on the ground. Feet should be shoulder-width apart.

2. Squeeze your thighs, bringing your knees together. Your feet should not move.

3. Now squeeze them apart to your starting position. Place your hands on the outside of your thighs for added resistance.

4. Repeat squeezers 10 to 15 times.

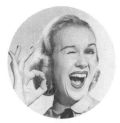

QUICK ⅆℬ PAINLESS

Check your posture! Whether you're exercising or not, a straight posture will do wonders for your back!

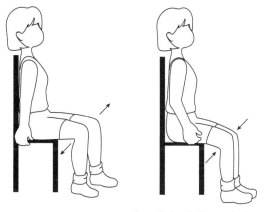

Figure 14.4: Squeezers: Not only will this help work those ab muscles, but all this moving around will help you maintain a better posture!

Leg Ups

1. Sit up straight with abdominals pulled in and feet planted firmly on the floor.

2. Extend your right leg so that it is straight out in front of you. Concentrate on tightening your thigh as you lift your leg up.

3. Lower your leg back to its starting position. Then repeat again for 10 to 15 times.

4. Repeat the same process with your left leg.

5. Use ankle weights to increase the resistance.

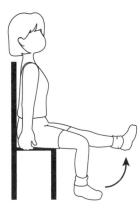

Figure 14.5: Leg Ups: Do this while you're typing a letter and keep the blood flowing!

Butt Tucks

1. Sit up straight in your chair.

2. Breathe in, filling up your diaphragm (your middle should expand).

3. Now, forcefully blow all of your air out, pulling your belly button into your spine. If you are doing this correctly, it will make your hips tilt up slightly.

4. Repeat this breathing in and out process 20 times.

YOU'LL THANK YOURSELF LATER

What a shocking idea! Your arms and knees should always (unless otherwise specified) be slightly bent. Think of these joints as the shock absorbers for your body. It will lighten your load and lessen the strain on your body.

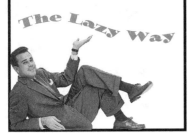

Congratulations! You've mastered the Pull Down exercise! Now, pull down a good movie and relax!

The Lazy Way

Pull Downs

1. You will need a dyna band or some elastic tubing for this exercise.

2. Sit up straight and extend your arms straight in front of you, holding the elastic tubing at forehead level. Hands should be a little less than a foot apart from each other.

3. Pull the band down toward your chest, squeezing your shoulder blades together. The distance between your hands will widen as your arms come down.

4. Return to your starting position and repeat 10 to 15 times.

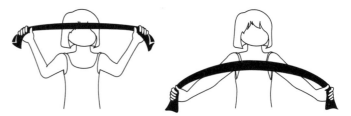

Figure 14.6: Pull Downs: Stuck on a creative problem at work? Do this exercise while musing on the latest question!

Pull Aparts

1. You can use dumbbells or elastic tubing to increase the resistance of this exercise.

2. Sit up straight with abdominals pulled in and feet firmly planted on the floor.

3. Bring your arms straight out in front of you at chest level, palms placed together and pointed forward.

4. Keeping your arms straight (slightly bent at elbows) start pulling them away from each other.

5. As you bring them backward, squeeze your shoulder blades together. This will push your chest out.

6. Return to your starting position and repeat 10 to 15 times.

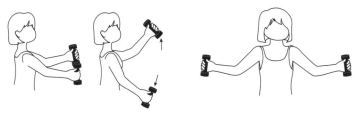

Figure 14.7: Pull Aparts: This is a great one for the lunch break . . . after sitting all morning, take some time to stretch out the upper body!

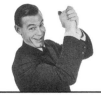

YOU'LL THANK YOURSELF LATER

Tool time. Keep a spare set of "tools" (dyna band, hand weights) at work to aid in your chair calisthenics. You can slip them into your drawer and grab them for break time or down time. Your co-workers will be impressed by your energy and efficiency. You might even encourage a friend to join you.

Press Ups

1. Place your palms on the arms of your chair and extend your arms until they are straight (keep a slight bend at your elbows), lifting yourself off the chair.

2. Hold this position for a count of three and then slowly lower yourself until you are sitting.

3. Repeat this process 10 times.

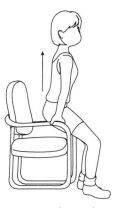

Figure 14.8: Press Ups: Try this in the morning when you first sit down to work, it'll get your blood flowing!

Chicken Wings

1. Sit up straight and hold two light dumbbells on your thighs. Your arms should be bent to form right angles.

2. Start lifting your arms up, keeping the right angles and your forearms parallel to the floor.

3. Raise arms to shoulder height, keeping your neck and upper back relaxed.

4. Slowly lower arms back down to your thighs and repeat 10 to 12 times.

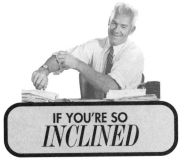

IF YOU'RE SO
INCLINED

Doing some quick exercises in the morning will get you going faster than a cup of coffee—give it a try!

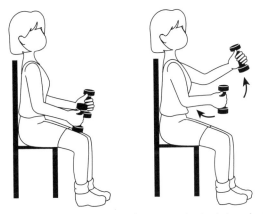

Figure 14.9: Chicken Wings: This may take both hands, but it's only a few minutes out of your day!

Bell Hoppers

1. Sit up straight, pulling abdominals in, and holding a dumbbell at your side.

2. Slowly shrug the shoulder upward on the side with the dumbbell. Keep your arms straight. (Movement resembles picking up a suitcase.)

3. Hold for a count of three then slowly lower your shoulder back down.

4. Repeat 10 to 15 times then do the same process with the other arm.

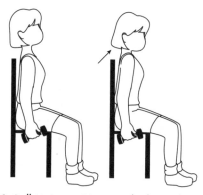

Figure 14.10: Bell Hoppers: You can do this with one arm and still have the other hand free to talk on the phone!

Congratulations! You've learned how to get fit while you sit! Treat yourself to a walk in the park and enjoy some fresh air!

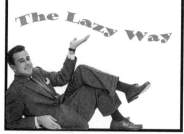

Rotators

1. Sit up straight, holding a dumbbell on your right thigh. Your arm should be bent to form a right angle.

2. Keeping your right elbow next to your side, start moving your arm outward. Your forearm should stay parallel to the floor.

3. Rotate your right arm as far as it will go without your elbow leaving your side.

4. Bring your arm slowly back to the starting position and repeat 10 to 12 times.

5. Repeat the same process with your left arm.

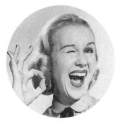

QUICK ⬭ PAINLESS

Waiting in the kitchen for water to boil? Grab a big can of soup and do a couple of Rotators while you wait!

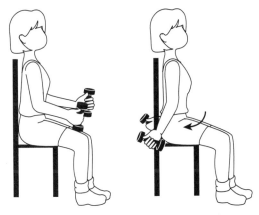

Figure 14.11: Rotators: Use this exercise to work on your upper arm muscles effortlessly!

Getting Time on Your Side

	The Old Way	The Lazy Way
Getting your exercises done	Who's got time?	At the office!
Working those abs	2 hours a week at the gym	5 minutes a day at the office
Working leg muscles	2 hours a week at the gym	5 minutes a day at the office
Working arm muscles	2 hours a week at the gym	5 minutes a day at the office
Working thigh muscles	2 hours a week at the gym	5 minutes a day at the office
Working upper arm muscles	2 hours a week at the gym	5 minutes a day at the office

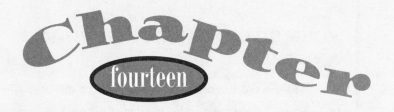

Hocus Pocus, Find Your Focus

Okay. **This time you know you can do it. You've made up your mind that you can live without chocolate. After all, the 2-pound bag of M&Ms you ate yesterday should last you a lifetime. A couple of days go by and you've managed to melt chocolate away from your memory. That is until you see the little Girl Scout coming to your door with cookies.**

As you munch on your Thin Mints, you wonder why it's so hard to stick to your goals. The truth is we make this whole goal business tough on ourselves. But, it doesn't have to be that way. Setting and accomplishing your goals does not require magic. It just takes a tiny push in the right direction. And, it so happens we're here to lend a hand.

In this chapter, we'll give you some simple tips to help you set your goals. Then we'll show you some guidelines for keeping your eating, exercise, and attitude in focus. So, put down your cookies and find out just how easy it is to reach your goals.

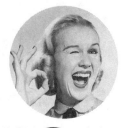

QUICK n PAINLESS

Give yourself bite size ("do" able) chunks of exercise throughout your day.

YOUR GOALS CAN BE SET WITHOUT ANY FRET

We all know we need to have goals. After all, they give us a sense of purpose and keep us motivated. But, there's a more important thing that goals can give you, and that's a sense of accomplishment when you achieve them. Yet, many of us don't know what this feels like because we set unrealistic goals (like living without chocolate).

The key to setting your goals is keeping them realistic. When you keep your goals "down-to-earth," you'll have purpose without any pressure. And, the best way to do this is to make them short, simple, lively, and flexible.

Keep It Short

Don't look at the whole mountain of pounds that you have in front of (or maybe behind) you. Rather, break up your long-term goals into shorter, more livable ones. It's quite okay to take baby steps. When you inch along you can be assured that you will keep going in the right direction. Short-term goals help you reach your peak without straining your will power.

Keep It Simple

When setting goals you want to avoid venturing into any gray areas. You won't get lost if you keep your goals black and white. In other words, be specific about what you want to do. Instead of pledging to "exercise more," decide on what activity you'll do, when you can do it, and how long you'll do it. Then all that's left is to just do it! The more specific your goals, the more simple they are to achieve.

Keep It Lively

The question is not "to be," but how will you become? The focus should not be on passive desires but on the actions that will take you to your desired goal. So, quit day-dreaming of how you'd like to be and concentrate on the lively acts that will get you there.

Keep It Flexible

If you set goals that are too rigid, you're liable to snap at some point (maybe when a Girl Scout comes knocking on your door!). Avoid depriving yourself or thinking in terms of "never" or "forever." You need to find some middle ground that bends with life's fluctuations. Flexible goals will ease you into healthier lifestyle changes.

TAKE AIM WITH YOUR KNIFE AND FORK

Healthy eating is the side of the weight-loss equation that usually takes the most struggle to succeed at. Mostly because we are constantly depriving ourselves in order to shed the pounds. This leads to the first guideline to help you focus on eating healthfully—never give up chocolate or any of your favorite (even decadent) foods! Here are some more pointers for hitting the center of balanced eating.

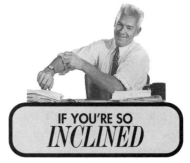

IF YOU'RE SO
INCLINED

Reality check. Divide up what types of exercise you need to perform to get fit. Make a workout plan and stick with it. If you're not improving in the appropriate areas after a month, vary it. Meet with a professional trainer to adjust or add variety to your plan.

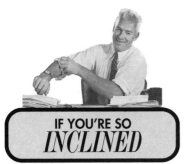

Variety is the spice of life. You don't have to be swinging single to enjoy a little change in your daily workout routine. It's useful to substitute or vary your workout schedule to keep it from becoming dull and dreary. If you're running on a tight schedule you may want to substitute the more vigorous, less time-consuming exercises (running steps) and more lengthy exercises (yoga) on days when your schedule permits.

- Concentrate on one food group at a time. Take a week to focus on how you can get in the recommended servings for each food group. When you are comfortable knowing what choices you can make for one food group then move on to the next one.

- Make mini-goals to lower the fat in your diet. For example, you can start by using a spray bottle instead of free-pouring, or you may decide not to butter your toast. Make small changes that won't leave you longing for fat.

- Eat more slowly. Put your fork down or drink some water between bites. Try not to be the first one to polish off the meal.

- Figure out how you can get all of your water in during the day. Start your morning off with a glass of water and drink one before you go to bed. That's two down—how will you get in the other six?

- Decide to eat only half of what's on your plate. Or, at least try to leave something behind. This will help you cut back on your portions especially when you are dining out.

- Slowly cut back on the sodas. Try other beverages like herbal teas or carbonated waters with an essence of fruit but no added sugars or sweeteners. Once you've cut back on sodas, target other processed foods you can eliminate.

- Allow yourself one or two indulgences a week. If you need more than that, you'll have to burn off the extra calories.

MAKE YOUR MARK WITH MOVEMENT

It's so important to stay focused on exercise because you have to do it for the rest of your life. Yikes! This is a scary thought, probably because we push ourselves too hard or consider it a form of punishment. But, we've shown you how you can exercise *The Lazy Way*—no pain, no hassle, no sweat (well, barely any), and you can still reap the benefits! Now we'll show you how to keep moving toward your mark.

- Schedule your exercise time in your planner/calendar at the beginning of every week. View your exercise time as an appointment with yourself.

- Take a five-or 10-minute walk right after dinner. When dining out, walk around a few blocks before driving home.

- Try a new activity every season. When you've mastered it you can move on to something else.

- Promise yourself that you will get out in nature at least once a month.

- Always remember to start gradually and build up slowly. You'll be doing this for the rest of your life so you might as well take your time.

- Find a buddy to exercise with. Whether it's a personal trainer, friend, club member, or your spouse, make it a habit to have a workout partner.

- Each week think of one way you can be more active and incorporate it into your lifestyle. For instance,

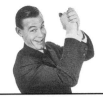

YOU'LL THANK YOURSELF LATER

Use it to lose it! Create a chart that shows how long you need to work out (select the activity of your choice) to burn up the fat and calories gained from your favorite foods eaten. For example, one order of small fries equals 20 minutes on the treadmill. You'll use up energy making the chart and you will have a better understanding of how much you need to move it to lose it! You may want to look back at the table at the end of Chapter 12 to help you figure out how to beat that treat!

park your car farther away or lose your remote control.

MENTAL MANEUVERS TO GET ON TARGET

Reaching your eating and exercise goals will happen only with the right frame of mind. You'll have to make some mental maneuvers to get on target. Follow this protocol to help you engage your attitude.

- Don't focus on how many pounds you want to shed. Instead, concentrate on the changes you make with your eating and exercise. Think "I will do," not "I will be."

- View your pound shedding as a process rather than another diet project. When making changes you need to ask yourself if you can eat or live that way for the rest of your life.

- Figure out what will work for you. How you shed your pounds will be as individual as you are.

- Forget about daily weighing. The scale is not the best way to monitor your progress. Instead, measure yourself every four to six weeks.

- Build your commitment. There are different levels of commitment: commitments you mentally make to yourself, commitments you make to yourself in writing, and commitments that you make to others. The latter is the most powerful form, the one you'll least likely break. That's why it's important to share your goals with other people.

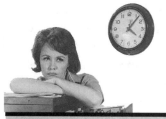

A COMPLETE WASTE OF TIME

The 3 Worst Ways to Work Out:

1. Not work out at all one week and then go at it every day the next.

2. Work out so hard one day that you can't move the next day (build up slowly).

3. Skip a workout because it didn't fit into your usual a.m. or p.m. slot (fit your exercise in where it works best for that day).

- Keep yourself motivated. Whether it's a pair of old jeans, an inspirational quote, a fresh goal, or a picture of you back in the good ol' days, place these items where they are visible. They'll fill you with enthusiasm every time you pass by them.

- Stay positive. Looking on the bright side will help lessen your load and loosen you up. Just turn the page and we'll give you a bunch of ways to keep your thoughts positive.

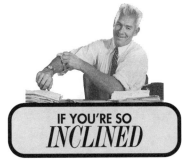

IF YOU'RE SO
INCLINED

In the beginning there was . . . you. Take a picture of yourself from your youth, high school years, college days, or young adulthood and place it on your bathroom mirror for encouragement. Do you want to look like that again or never again? Use it to inspire you to keep up your newfound and easy-to-maintain healthy values.

Getting Time on Your Side

	The Old Way	The Lazy Way
Setting your goals	Years and years	Daily, weekly, monthly
Working toward your goals	Years and years	Daily, weekly, monthly
Reaching your goals	Years and years	Daily, weekly, monthly
Feeling better about yourself	Years and years	Daily, weekly, monthly
Seeing a difference	Years and years	Daily, weekly, monthly
Getting upset with yourself for not reaching your goals	Every day	Never again

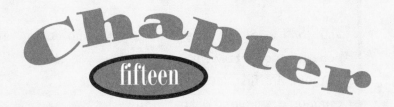

Make Your Own Mental Magic

It's one of life's many mysteries . . . where does the little voice live inside your head? And how come it's never quiet? (Talk about a workout!) It bounces around flashing new cognitions, while other times it plays the same old tapes. Well, there are some things we just don't know the answer to, but we do know that what your little voice tells you determines how successful you will be at shedding your pounds.

The magical thing is that you can control what your little voice says. It can be as easy as the stroke of a wand to make your negative thoughts disappear. Then you can fill your hat with positive ones. Take a look at these tricks and treats to help you (and your little voice) stay upbeat.

NUKE YOUR NEGATIVE THOUGHTS

Negative thoughts are one of the key factors that can undermine your pound shedding ability. These statements (which are usually false) only set you up for failure. Since we know

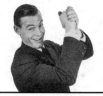

P.S. I love you! Take a moment each morning to jot down three positive statements about yourself. Keep them all in a notebook, and when you're feeling blue or discouraged flip through for a quick mental hug.

you don't want to waste precious time and energy on negative thoughts, we'll show you how you can get rid of them. But first, let's take a look at some of the most common detrimental deliberations.

- The infamous, "I can't!" If you think you can't do something, you probably won't. Realize that anything and everything is possible, and you can do whatever you set your mind to.

- The notion that you "should" always clean your plate or you "should" never refuse food offerings can sabotage your eating. Shy away from this rigid thinking. Rather, eat when you're hungry and stop before you're full.

- When you make excuses, you allow yourself to continue bad eating habits. It's amazing how we can rationalize anything to suit our fancy . . . "Oh, just one little piece won't hurt" . . . "That piece was so little, I could have another one" . . . "Well, I'll take just one more piece because who knows when I'll have this chance again" . . .

- Then comes the self-defeating thoughts . . . "I'm just a big, fat pig!" Putting yourself down only fuels the vicious negative cycle. After all, since you're a pig you better eat the whole thing, right?!

- Judging your foods as "good" or "bad" can encourage the wrong kind of thinking and eating. Telling yourself you can't have a food because it's "bad," makes you want it all the more. Your little voice will argue between "never" and "gotta have it."

Healthy eating is not about "good" or "bad" foods; it's about making choices and using moderation.

■ How many times have you let the scale decide how your day will be? We've already told you how unreliable the scale can be. Don't let it have any power over you. The best way to avoid being a slave to the scale is by focusing on your habits instead of the weight.

So, how do you nuke these negative thoughts? You need to stop them in their tracks! You must consciously halt them before they flatten you. It's pretty easy—all you have to do is say "STOP!" Whether you do this with your inner voice or you shout it with your own, saying "STOP" will interrupt this negative flow. It takes a little practice, but you'll get the hang of it in no time.

POOF! INSTANT POSITIVE THOUGHTS

■ The most effective way to challenge your negative thoughts is to think of your accomplishments. Reflecting on these positive achievements will give you greater self-confidence and self-control.

■ Focus on your goals. Think about the reasons why you want to lose weight or change your behavior and how you will feel when you get there.

■ Concentrate on long-term results rather than short-term pleasures. Ask yourself if you really need that piece of cake. If you really do, then have it, but most of the time you'll find you don't.

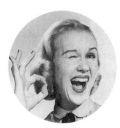

QUICK ⬭ PAINLESS

Change, change, change! It does you good. People are naturally resistant to change. But truth or consequences—what feels better? Sticking with your old, bad habits or trying on some new ones for size?

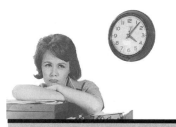

A COMPLETE WASTE OF TIME

The 3 Worst Ways You Can Sabotage Your Weight Loss Plans/Goals Are:

1. To give up after a difficult day of exercise and eating.

2. To let other people's negative opinions matter to you.

3. To physically put forth the effort but to mentally brow beat yourself.

It's a complete waste of time to keep thinking of yourself in a negative light.

- When faced with making a difficult choice ask yourself, "How will I feel after I eat it?" Often foods that look tempting are not that satisfying. Remember that nothing tastes as good as being fit feels.

- Forget about any past failures at shedding your pounds. Glean from these attempts what worked for you and let go of the rest.

- Surround yourself with inspirational quotes an sayings. They'll lift your spirits and help motivate you to achieve your goals.

- Let your little voice give you "pats on the back." Always acknowledge your triumphs no matter how big or small.

You'll know you're making progress when your positive thoughts outweigh your negative ones. You can get a jump-start on making your own mental magic by creating a list of positive affirmations that you can repeat to yourself. These statements can reflect your accomplishments, goals, or reasons why "you're worth it." (You are worth it, you know!) In the morning (after you brush your teeth) stand before a mirror and repeat your affirmations to yourself. Whenever you feel yourself slipping toward negative thinking, get out your list and be positive. You'll come to believe in yourself more and more.

WHAT YOU SEE IS WHAT YOU GET

Another aspect of staying sanguine is creating images in addition to your positive thoughts. This is done by visualizing—thinking in pictures rather than words. Imagine how it will feel to be in the clothes' size of your dreams (of course, we mean your realistic dreams). What are you wearing? What color is it? How many compliments are you receiving? When you visualize scenarios like this you reinforce your commitment and enhance your positive thinking.

Visualization can also be used to turn negative images to your advantage. For instance, if every time you saw a doughnut you imagined cellulite on your thighs, it would be a lot easier to pass it up. However you decide to use it, visualization is a powerful tool for you to create your own mental magic.

ALL THESE TRICKS DESERVE A TREAT

A sure way to stay on track is to reward yourself for every step you make in the right direction. You need to pat yourself on the back and what better way is there than by rewarding yourself. Here is a list of treats for the tricks you will master to make your pounds disappear. Add your own special delights, but make sure they are non-food related.

- Treat yourself to a massage.
- Enjoy a luxurious bubble bath.
- Buy a bouquet of flowers.
- Read a good book.
- Sign up for a class you've always wanted to take.
- Purchase a new outfit.
- Write yourself a congratulatory note.

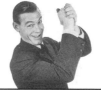

YOU'LL THANK YOURSELF LATER

It's habit forming! Make it a habit to state your personal weight loss/ health goals to yourself each morning as you brush your teeth. Uttering these positive statements daily helps to internalize your weight loss goals until they become second nature.

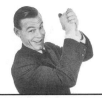

Don't worry. Be happy! You've made changes in your eating and exercise. It's time now to revamp your mental image of your physical self. Stop concentrating on your negatives and start focusing on your positives. You have beautiful eyes, you are tall, and your skin glows! Find your best qualities and write them down. Say them each morning to incorporate them into your self-image.

▪ Get a facial or a manicure.

▪ Go for a night out on the town.

▪ Rent your favorite movie.

Creating your own mental magic is knowing how to quiet your little voice when it wants to be negative. It's knowing how to persuade it to be positive. And the magic truly begins when you allow this little voice to sing your praises! Don't forget—you're worth it!

Getting Time on Your Side

	The Old Way	The Lazy Way
Getting rid of negative thoughts	Never	In a flash
Filling up on positive thoughts	Rarely	In an instant
Visualizing your thoughts	Occasionally (so many years of wasted time!)	In a blink
Time spent saying "I can't"	Years	Never again
Time spent listening to negative thoughts	A lifetime	Never again
Time spent realizing you're worth it!	Never	Every minute, every day!

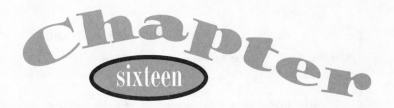

The Quick Switch

It's a logical sequence. First you make the habit, then the habit makes you. The problem lies in your habit making more of you than you want. That's when you have to put your foot down (it actually feels better if you put both feet down), and figure out a way to change your behavior.

Changing your habits can be a difficult process, but not if you do it *The Lazy Way*. You just need to follow a few simple steps to make your bad habits disappear. The first step is awareness. The second one is substitution. Then all you have to do is practice. You'll see how these strategies will help you make the quick switch in no time at all.

CAUTION! BE AWARE! HABITS ARE FORMING EVERYWHERE

Have you ever had the smell of fresh baked goods lure you into a bakery? Do you always buy popcorn when you go to the movies? Have you ever stared blindly into the refrigerator? These are examples of eating triggers. They are events or stimuli that can often lead to poor eating habits. Sometimes they

Stop, look, and listen. Make yourself account- able by keeping track of everything (and how much of it) you put in your mouth for a few days. Awareness is half the battle. Remember to stop and think about why you're eating, to look at the portion size of what you're eating, and listen to your stom- ach to let you know when you're full and not just eating to fill another need.

involve your senses (smell, sight, sound), while other times they center around your moods or emotions (anger, boredom, anxiety, etc.).

The first thing you need to do is become aware of what triggers you to eat poorly so that you can take these undesirable habits and replace them with new, healthy ones. When you open the refrigerator, you need to ask yourself, "Why am I doing this? Am I truly hungry?"

Here are some common situations involving poor eating behavior. See which ones you can identify with and ask yourself what it is that makes them a problem for you.

- You eat to feel better when you're unhappy, bored, or tense.
- You wake up in the middle of the night and head to the kitchen for a snack.
- You munch on different foods because you are avoiding a task.
- You reward yourself with food after completing a task.
- You eat because it's mealtime, even if you're not hungry.
- You eat more than you normally would because you're watching television.
- You clean out the cupboards when you're alone and lonely.
- You taste more food while cooking dinner than you eat when you sit down for dinner.

- You always "pig-out" at social gatherings.
- You feel compelled to clean your plate and eat the kids' leftovers.

These scenarios will hopefully make you aware of food habits you may need to switch. Be sure to add any other situations that are specific to you. Once you are aware of your unhealthy eating habits you are ready to move on to the next step—substituting healthy eating habits in their place.

THE EASY SWITCHAROO— MAKE IT WORK FOR YOU

Just as you say, "STOP!" to your negative thoughts, it also helps to interrupt your bad habits. Then you can replace them with positive, healthy ones. The alternative desirable habits are actions or activities you can do. The more mentally and physically you can become involved (don't go overboard though) and the longer the action/activity lasts, the more effectively it will stave off undesirable behaviors.

You can make substitution work better if you determine, ahead of time, several substitute actions. One way to do this is to have a list of alternatives prepared for the times when you are tempted. That way, at any moment of temptation, you'll have some satisfying options available. Here are some suggestions. Be sure to add substitutions of your own that will give you satisfaction and enjoyment.

Bravo! You've orchestrated your workout regimen so it plays in harmony with your new eating patterns. That's music to our ears! Give yourself a standing ovation and then take a bow (you just added a stretch to your workout), you deserve it!

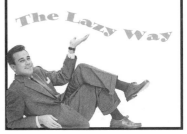

The Lazy Way

- Go for a walk.

- Go shopping.

- Call a friend.

- Brush your teeth.

- Pick up a hobby.

- Drink some water.

- Read a book.

- Take a bubble bath.

- Make yourself some hot herbal tea.

- Meditate.

PRACTICE THAT'S PRACTICALLY PAINLESS

The final step to behavior change is lots of practice. Even though this is an easy part, it can be frustrating because it takes time for your habits to change. So, give yourself a month or two and practice one thing at a time. Just be aware and substitute over and over again until your new habits become a natural part of your every day life.

Practice can also serve as a recovery plan when you feel like you've gone off track. Sometimes you can have a bad day, which is okay since what counts is consistency and not an occasional slip. But if your slip has turned into a sprawling fall you can follow these tips to pick yourself back up.

- Clear your mind of any guilt or negative thoughts.

- Review your goals and positive statements.

Substitute/schedule a massage for your workout one day. Not only does it feel good but your muscles are still being moved . . . this is the ultimate *Lazy Way* you benefit without lifting a finger (or toe).

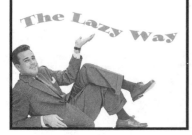

The Lazy Way

- Reflect on the undesirable behaviors that you were unable to substitute. Review your substitution list and decide which activity you will do the next time the same situation occurs.

- Get back on your regular eating and exercise schedule.

- Practice, practice, practice!

DROP YOURSELF A LINE AND YOU'LL KNOW YOU'RE DOING FINE

One of the best ways to stay in touch with your eating, exercise, and attitude is to keep a journal. A journal can teach you about your thoughts and feelings. It can show you why and when you eat due to emotions or stress. It can help you view each day as a new and separate challenge. And, it becomes a record of your life-changing process.

You can write down whatever your little heart desires in your journal. It's up to you how long or short your entries are. The important thing is that you turn to your journal for daily renewal. Here are some suggestions for making the most of your journal-keeping.

- State your goals and what you'll do to work toward them. These can be daily, weekly, or monthly goals.

- Record your list of positive statements about yourself and your life. Review this list every day and keep adding to it as you come up with more affirmations.

- Keep your list of substitutions on a certain page, handy for the times when you may be tempted.

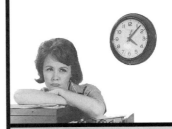

A COMPLETE WASTE OF TIME

The 3 Worst Things You Can Do While Making Changes for a Healthier, Happier You:

1. Let others dissuade or discourage you.

2. Let indecision creep in.

3. Let your momentum slow down.

- Write down your thoughts and feelings regarding life, food, exercise, and anything else you desire.

- Don't forget to record your set-backs. Use them as experiences to learn from.

- Put a copy of your favorite inspirational quotes, sayings, or prayers to keep you motivated.

- Record the good things that happen during your day. What did you like best? What would you do differently next time?

- Keep a log of your eating and exercising. Focus on your number of fat grams and food servings, your water intake, and how many minutes you exercised.

- One check ahead! If recording all the details in your journal is too time-consuming, try checking it off on a chart instead. Track your exercise, fat grams, food servings, and water intake. Stick the chart on your refrigerator or put it in your day planner. Make sure to make multiple copies to grab as needed.

- In addition to tracking your food, write down the time and how you feel as you're eating. This will give you an idea of your eating patterns and challenges.

- Save a spot for your measurements. Record them every four to six weeks and be sure to put down an inches and pounds list.

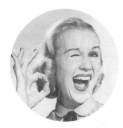

QUICK **n** PAINLESS

Put your journal objectives on post-it notes and place them in several strategic places. You might post one on your refrigerator, one in your wallet, and another on the dashboard of your car. These little yellow flags will keep you attuned to attaining your goals.

- Use stickers to give you an extra boost of confidence on the days you stay on track.

- Don't forget your reward list. And, every time you switch undesirable behaviors for alternative desirable ones, be sure to treat yourself.

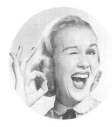

QUICK ⓝ PAINLESS

What's good for the goose is good for the gander. Try this with your mate or a friend. Ask them to list their top three favorite physical attributes for you and you do the same for them. You'll be surprised and delighted how special you look through another's eyes.

Getting Time on Your Side

	The Old Way	The Lazy Way
Breaking bad habits	Never	The second you're aware
Substituting good habits	Never	A month or two
Practicing new habits	Never (so many years of wasted time!)	A little time each day
Being led by your food triggers	All day	Never again
Using food to feel better	Every day	Not anymore!
Feeling guilty	Every minute	Never again!

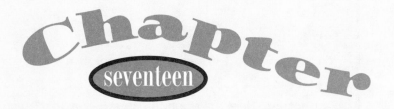

seventeen

Create an Illusion

Imagine getting all the right curves with none of the sweat. No, you're not going in for liposuction. And, you don't have to wire your jaws shut. You can reshape your body in the laziest of ways with your clothes!

In this chapter, we'll outfit you with several clothing tips to help you lose inches instantly. You'll know how to dress best for your body type. You'll also find out sneaky ways to sculpt those inches off, from undergarments to accessories. So get ready for the bare necessities.

THE BARE TRUTH ON BODY TYPES

You're pretty much stuck in the body you were born with. This can be good or bad news, but either way you need to embrace your shape (whatever shape it's in!). When you know your body type you can figure out what clothes will look best on you. Let's look at some common shapes and their complementary "shape-ups."

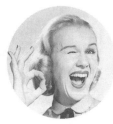

Top Heavy

You know you're top heavy if you look like an upside-down pear. Your top is substantially broader/bigger than your bottom. Here are some tips to even the load.

- Wear a darker color on top to minimize and a lighter color on the bottom to maximize (or balance).

- Stay away from boxy shapes (i.e., shoulder pads) that will accentuate your upper body.

- Choose flowing layers that disguise rather than tight or fitted clothes that will emphasize your "over-endowed" areas.

- Draw the eye down. Stay away from horizontal lines, busy prints, and lots of fussy details (breast pockets, excessive buttons, added flourishes).

- Whatever your proportions, remember to accentuate your positives. If you are bigger on top and have a smaller bottom half, try wearing sleek, body slimming bottoms (leggings or a narrow skirt for women, fitted slacks and trousers for men) with an oversized tunic or jersey on top.

Bottom Heavy

You know you're bottom heavy if your body resembles an upright pear shape. Your bottom half is substantially wider/bigger than your upper region. Here are some tricks to help balance you out.

- Use color selection to mask your middle/bottom. Choose darker colors to conceal your lower regions and lighter ones to emphasize your upper regions.

- Use shoulder pads to your advantage. Find tops and jackets that have a more defined shoulder line to balance your top against your bottom.

- Adding layers can disguise your problem area. If you have a small upper body and waist with a bigger bottom try tucking in a blouse and adding a longer, hip-length blazer.

- Keep your bottom half all one color. Match your skirt/slacks to your stockings and to your shoes. Wearing all one tone keeps the eyes going down.

- Keep it simple! A dark suit and crisp shirt without fussy details and clashing patterns will make the most of what you've got (and hide what you don't want to show!).

- Find your length and stick with it. If you have a heavy bottom, thighs, and calves, go maxi (mid-ankle). If you just have a heavy bottom and thighs, go mid-length (mid-thigh). If you only have a heavy bottom and good legs, go mini (mid-thigh).

The Long and the Short of It

This may be carrying the fruit analogy too far, but think of pineapples and oranges. If you are tall and ample or short and ample it's hard to disguise your shape without thinking of a drape. But you need a little definition in your designs to keep you from feeling like and looking

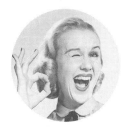

QUICK ⟨IP⟩ PAINLESS

Don't forget that nothing is more forgiving than black. Slim your wardrobe and your bottom line with an ample supply of black skirts, slacks, and leggings.

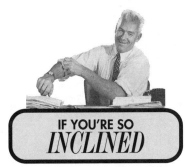

Take advantage of the fact that you can always make something smaller and shorter but it is much harder to make it larger and longer. If you find a piece of clothing that is the perfect color and style but a tad too large or long, have it altered to fit you perfectly. It's as good as having it made for you, and you don't even have to start from scratch.

like an overgrown bed sheet. Here are some tips to take advantage of your height or lack of it.

- Use your height to your full advantage—show off long legs with a well-placed slit in your skirt, show off a long neck with a lower cut décolletage.

- When you're tall, you can get away with daring accessories that a shorter person couldn't carry off. Drape a dramatic shawl over your shoulders or add a long strand of beads to an otherwise simple, yet elegant monochromatic outfit.

- If you are a person of smaller stature, the length of your sleeves, hem lines, and cuffs is very important. If they fit your width but are too long for your height, have them tailored to fit your proper proportions.

- Use catalogs to your advantage. Depending on your stature, shop from catalogs that carry larger/taller sizes or sizes for people 5'5" and under.

- If you're vertically challenged, make the most of your height by adding to it! Invest in some quality, comfortable higher heels that will lengthen your leg and will give your body a more linear look.

RESHAPING YOUR FOUNDATION

There is so much you can do nowadays to reshape your body. Whether you want to boost your bust, trim your thighs, or tuck your tummy, the secret is in your foundation. Here's how you can use various undergarments to your advantage. The great thing is no one has to know what goes on behind closed drawers.

Don't Bust Out

Here are tips for purchasing the correct bra for your size. Get fitted for your bra by a "fit specialist" in a department store. Go for wider, padded strap that won't gouge. If spilling over is a problem, try on one cup size larger. Find a brand that makes deeper cups if the center of your bra is not laying flat on your breast bone. If you're well endowed, use underwire style for firmer support.

If at first you don't succeed, try on and on again. Just because you were a 38 DD in one brand doesn't mean you'll be the same size in a bra by a different designer. Don't go strictly by tag sizes; you'll find it's liberating to forget about size and go for fit, comfort, and style! And when you find one that works, buy a few.

Create Some Curves with Corsets

Full-body briefers or corsets look pretty and make you feel beautiful. With this single garment you can tame your tummy and whittle your waist.

Slip Into Sleekness

When the look you're going for is a sexy silhouette under a body skimming dress, try a body slimmer. It's a firming slip that will pinch in the fat without giving you the squeeze. A good rule of thumb (or thigh) for fitting a body shaper is to bring along a knit dress or other tight

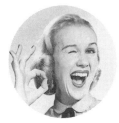

QUICK ɪɴ PAINLESS

It's a bum wrap (and tummy too)! Whittle your waist and tuck your tummy without ever stepping in a doctor's door. With a few simple undergarments, such as waist cinchers and body briefers, you can make the inches disappear in a cinch.

fitting garment to try on the body toner with. It'll save you from returning again and again.

Shrink Yourself with Stockings

Lose an inch without the pinch! There are a variety of hose that can hold you in without hugging you too tight. Check the packaging labels that explain the levels of hold (light, medium, and extra). Some of these super powerful control top hose can make you seem 5 to 10 pounds lighter!

ALL TOGGED OUT WITH THE TRICKS OF THE TRADE

There's more to dressing slim than merely reshaping your foundation. You can't forget the outer layers. Here's a closet full of tips and tricks to shrink you down even more.

- Make sure your clothes fit you properly. Clothes that are too tight, short, or binding can give you the appearance of looking larger than you are. Clothes that are too baggy or loose can make you look bigger too.

- Have a seamstress make a few basics for you. The cost may be more up front, but in the long run you'll save yourself time, energy, and money searching everywhere for your perfect fit.

- Quality fabric, simple designs, and a few well-placed touches can make you instantly as beautiful outside as you are within.

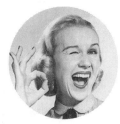

- Have your colors done professionally. Wearing the right shade (especially near your face) can lighten and brighten your looks. Then you can weed out the duds from your chest.

- For a leaner, trimmer line, look for such shaping details as vertical darts and princess seams. The tailoring helps to present a more polished (thinner) picture. If there aren't any of these features and there is ample room to insert them, have a seamstress add them to the garment.

- Basic black—it's a classic! It looks good on nearly everyone and should be an essential in your closet. Black is slimming, timeless, and suitable for all seasons. If you buy some key pieces in a multi-season fabric, it can carry you through the year. Besides, you never know when you might be in need of that little black dress.

- Go for the monochromatic presentation. Choose your preferred color and use it as your signature shade. Using just one color (or different intensities of one shade) will give your appearance a longer, leaner look. Tie in your accessories (shoes, stocking, handbag) by having them in the same tone.

- Remember to choose clothes that flatter your body type. Accentuate the good and cover the bad.

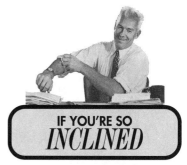

IF YOU'RE SO
INCLINED

In a color rut? Have your colors done by a professional to see what looks best on you. Your eyes and your wardrobe will be opened to a whole new spectrum of shades.

THE ACCENT IS ON ACCESSORIES

Even the smallest details matter when you're slimming down your appearance. Choosing the right accessories

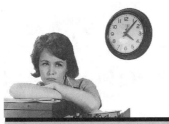

The 3 Worst Things You Can Do When Accessorizing:

1. Pull together an elegant, simply designed ensemble and then clutter it up with too much jewelry . . . remember to keep it simple.

2. Pull together a mono-chromatic outfit and then wear shoes, stockings, and a hand-bag that stand out more than the clothes.

3. Pull together a great look and then have your hair look out of date and in need of a trim.

will help you complete the illusion. Follow these tips to accentuate your best features, from your toenails to your topknot.

- Avoid chokers. Choose longer necklaces that will draw your eyes down.

- Spend some time at a cosmetics counter and have your make-up done by a professional. They can show you how to lift your cheek bones with just a little foundation and blush.

- When you have your colors done, you can find out which precious metal looks best with your coloring. Stick to jewelry with the metal that makes you sparkle most.

- Getting a tan can give your limbs a faux tone-up, but you should avoid lying out in the sun. Go for a fake tan instead and use some self-tanning lotion.

- Get a professional hair stylist to give you the most flattering cut for you face shape and lifestyle.

- For an instant face-lift, pull your hair up, back, and away from your face. French twists, chignons, and braids are simple, sophisticated styles that will do the trick.

- Pay attention to the smallest of details by maintaining your nails from your fingertips to your toes. This will let you put your best foot and hand forward.

Getting Time on Your Side

	The Old Way	The Lazy Way
Boosting your bust	Hours	Half a minute
Trimming your thighs	Weeks	Half a minute
Tucking your tummy	Months	Half a minute (and lots of sweat!)
Figuring out what to wear	Hours	A few minutes
Making do with things that almost fit	Years	Never again!
Dealing with colors	Hours	2 seconds

More Lazy Stuff

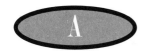

A

How to Get Someone Else to Do It

YOUR EATING

- American Diabetes Association (call local chapter for info)
- American Dietetic Association (800) 366-1655
- American Heart Association (800) 242-8721
- Center for Human Nutrition (402) 559-5500
- Duke University Diet and Fitness Program (800) 362-8446
- Hospitals (in-house weight-loss/eating programs)
- Johns Hopkins Weight Management Center (410) 550-2330
- Registered Dietitians
- Stanford Weight Loss Risk and Reduction Program, Stanford University (415) 723-5868
- Weight Control Center—New York Hospital (212) 583-1000
- Weight Watchers International (800) 651-6000

YOUR EXERCISE

- Aerobics and Fitness Association of America (800) 365-5376
- American College of Sports Medicine (317) 637-9200
- American Council on Exercise (800) 529-8277
- American Running and Fitness Association (800) 776-2732
- City Recreation Department
- Cooper Fitness Center
- International Spa and Fitness Association
- Jazzercise (800) 348-4748
- Local health clubs
- National Academy of Sports Medicine
- National Federation of Personal Trainers (800) 729-6378
- National Strength and Conditioning Association
- Spri Performance Systems (800) 488-7774
- Women's Sports and Fitness Foundation
- YMCA/YWCA

YOUR ATTITUDE

- American Psychology Association
- Overeater's Anonymous
- Personal shoppers (Lane Bryant, Macy's, Nordstrom)
- Weight Watchers International (800) 651-6000

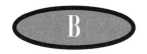

If You Really Want More, Read These

YOUR EATING

100% Pleasure, Nancy Baggett and Ruth Glick, Rodale Press, 1994.

The American Dietetic Association's Complete Food & Nutrition Guide, Roberta Larson Duyff, Chronimed Publishing, 1998.

The Art of Low Calorie Cooking, Sally Schneider, Stewart, Tabori and Chang, 1990.

Bowes & Church's Food Values of Portions Commonly Used, Jean Pennington, Lippincott–Raven Publishers, 1997.

The Complete and Up-to-date Fat Book, Karen J. Bellerson, Avery Publishing Group, 1993.

Cooking Light Cookbook, Nancy J. Fitzpatrick, Oxmoor House, 1996.

The Delicious! Collection: Simple Recipes for Healthy Living, Sue Frederick, Scb Distributors, 1992.

Eating Thin For Life, Anne Fletcher, Chapters Publishing, Ltd., 1997.

Exchange For All Occasions, Marion J. Franz, out of print.

Fast Food Facts, Marion J. Franz, Chronimed Publishing, 1997.

Graham Kerr's Minimax Cookbook, Graham Kerr, Perigee, 1994.

Great Good Food, Julee Rosso, Crown Publishing, 1993.

Lighter, Quicker, Better, Richard Sax and Marie Simmons, William Morrow and Co., 1995.

Low-Fat One-Dish Meals From Around the World, Jane Marsh Dieckmann, 1993, out of print.

The Mediterranean Kitchen, Joyce Goldstein, William Morrow and Co. Paper, 1998.

Moosewood Restaurant's Low-Fat Favorites, ed. Pam Krauss, Clarkson Potter, 1996.

New Dieter's Cook Book, Heidi McNutt, Better Homes and Gardens Books, 1997.

New Vegetarian Cuisine, Linda Rosensweig, Rodale Press, 1993.

Nutrition Action Healthletter.

Report of the Dietary Guidelines Advisory Committee on the Dietary Guidelines for Americans, U.S. Department of Agriculture.

Smart Cooking, Graham Kerr, Doubleday, 1991.

The Surgeon General's Report on Nutrition and Health, U.S. Department of Health and Human Services.

Tufts University Diet and Nutrition Letter.

The Tufts University Guide to Total Nutrition, Stanley Gershoff, HarperCollins Publishers, 1996.

YOUR EXERCISING

ACSM Fitness Book, ACSM, Human Kinetics Publishing, 1997.

Galloway's Book on Running, Jeff Galloway, Galloway Productions, 1984.

Living Fit magazine.

Men's Fitness magazine.

The New Aerobics for Women, Kenneth and Mildred Cooper, out of print.

Penn State Sports Medicine Newsletter.

Runner's World magazine.

Shape magazine.

Smart Exercise, Covert Bailey, Houghton Mifflin Co., 1996.

Walking magazine.

YOUR ATTITUDE

Codependent No More, Melody Beattie, Hazelden, 1996.

First Things First, Stephen Covey, Fireside, 1996.

Love Yourself Thin, Victoria Moran, Rodale Press, 1997.

Nothing Bad Happens Ever, Joan Fountain, Gold Leaf Press, 1997.

Personal Best, George Sheehan, Rodale Press, 1992.

The Power of 5, Dr. Harold H. Bloomfield and Dr. Robert K. Cooper, Rodale Press, 1996.

The Seven Habits of Highly Effective People, Stephen Covey, G.K. Hall & Co., 1997.

Something to Smile About, Zig Ziglar, Thomas Nelson, 1997.

You Can Heal Your Life, Louise L. Hay, Hay House, 1987.

YOUR POUND SHEDDING

Biomarkers, William Evans, Fireside, 1992.

Choose to Lose, Dr. Ron and Nancy Goor, Houghton Mifflin Co., 1995

The Complete Idiot's Guide to Losing Weight, Susan McQuillan with Dr. Edward Saltzman, Alpha Books, 1998.

Controlling Your Fat Tooth, Joseph C. Piscatella, Workman Publishing Company, 1991.

Eat More, Weigh Less, Dr. Dean Ornish, Harperperennial Library, 1994.

Eater's Choice, Dr. Ron and Nancy Goor, Houghton Mifflin Co., 1995.

Eating Thin for Life, Anne Fletcher, Chapters Publishing, Ltd., 1995.

Fat Chance: Your Best Chance For Permanent Weight Loss, Joan Cortopassi and Annette Cain, Alden Books, Stockton, CA, 1996.

The Fit or Fat Woman, Covert Bailey, Houghton Mifflin Co., 1989.

Making the Case for Yourself: A Diet Book for Smart Women, Susan Estrich, Putnam Publishing Group, 1998.

The New Fit or Fat, Covert Bailey, Houghton Mifflin Co., 1991.

Prevention magazine.

Strong Women Stay Slim, Miriam E. Nelson, Bantam Books, 1998.

The Undiet, Kim Jordan, Peanut Butter Publishing, 1997.

The Weight Control Digest.

Why Women Need Chocolate, Debra Waterhouse, Hyperion Press, 1995.

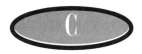

C

If You Don't Know What It Means/Does, Look Here

aerobic   In the presence of oxygen.

aerobic training   Continuous movement of the larger muscle groups of the body so that their need for oxygen is increased.

body shapers   Foundation garments constructed mostly of heavyweight nylon and lycra that smooth and hold your body's curves.

caloric deficit   A loss of energy created when your food energy (calories) is smaller than the total energy (calories) you use resulting in weight loss.

calorie   A unit of energy used to express the heat output of an organism and the fuel value of food.

eating triggers   Events or stimuli that often lead to poor eating habits. They can be external (senses) or internal (emotions, moods).

fiber   Also referred to as bulk or roughage, it is an indigestible material in human food that stimulates the intestine to peristalsis. Recommended daily intake is 25 to 30 grams.

free foods   Food items that have minimal calories and just a trace of fat (seasonings, condiments, herbs, flavorings, etc.).

hydrogenated fats Unsaturated fats that have been chemically processed to become thickened or more solid. Hydrogenated fats are therefore artificially saturated fats that are as bad for you as naturally saturated fats.

interval training While doing aerobic exercise you add intervals of speed or intensity to your normal pace (i.e., wind sprints). You can become fitter faster with interval training.

maximum heart rate The point at which your heart is beating at its maximum level; it can no longer increase its pumping.

metabolism The chemical changes in living cells by which energy is provided for vital processes and activities (i.e., lean mass energy requirements, digestion, exercise, daily activities).

monochromatic Having or consisting of one color or hue.

phytochemicals Chemical compounds found in foods of plant origin that have therapeutic/pharmacological properties (i.e., anti-cancer, anti-oxidant).

plateau The period of time when your weight remains at a certain level. Changing your exercise program (i.e., activity choices, frequency, intensity, duration) can help you come off a plateau.

resting heart rate The rate at which your heart beats when you are resting.

saturated fat (includes hydrogenated fat) The least desirable type of food fat. Saturated fats are often solids at room temperature. (Examples are butter, margarine, and lard.)

set point The constant weight at which your body has a tendency to remain. Lack of exercise, high-fat foods, overeating, and not eating enough (starvation) can raise your body's set point.

strength training Also called resistance training or weight lifting, this type of exercise forces muscles to work hard by introducing resistance to their movement. It can be done by using machines, free weights, elastic tubing, or the weight of your own body.

target heart rate Safe and efficient level of exertion (usually a range such as 65 percent to 80 percent of your maximum heart rate) where you may be breathing hard but you can speak easily.

thermogenesis The amount of calories burned digesting, absorbing, and utilizing food.

trans-free spreads Margarine products that are made with very little hydrogenation so they contain less saturated fat grams. The most popular trans-free spreads are made with canola oil.

whole grain An unprocessed, complex carbohydrate that contains fiber, vitamins, and minerals (brown rice, whole wheat, rye, oat, barley, whole grain cereals, etc.). At least half of your breads/cereals/grains servings should be whole grain.

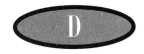

It's Time for Your Reward

Once You've Done This	Reward Yourself
Become aware of food triggers	Give yourself a hug
Completed your food journal	Give yourself a bouquet of flowers
Developed your treat list	Treat yourself to a treat
Developed your nonfood reward list	Choose a reward from the list
Gathered your exercise supplies	Pick up a new fitness outfit
Made your dumbbells	Give yourself a workout in nature
Made planned leftovers	Give yourself a night of no cooking
Placed your motivational items where you can see them	Give yourself a massage
Planned snack times	Get a new CD
Set your goals	Treat yourself to a night out

Where to Find What You're Looking For

Now you can do these tasks, too!

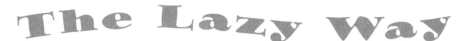

The Lazy Way

Starting to think there are a few more of life's little tasks that you've been putting off? Don't worry—we've got you covered. Take a look at all of *The Lazy Way* books available. Just imagine—you can do almost anything *The Lazy Way!*

Clean Your House The Lazy Way
By Barbara H. Durham
0-02-862649-4

Handle Your Money The Lazy Way
By Sarah Young Fisher and Carol Turkington
0-02-862632-X

Care for Your Home The Lazy Way
By Terry Meany
0-02-862646-X

Train Your Dog The Lazy Way
By Andrea Arden
0-87605180-8

Take Care of Your Car The Lazy Way
By Michael Kennedy and Carol Turkington
0-02-862647-8

Keep Your Kids Busy The Lazy Way
By Barbara Nielsen and Patrick Wallace
0-02-863013-0

*All Lazy Way books are just $12.95!

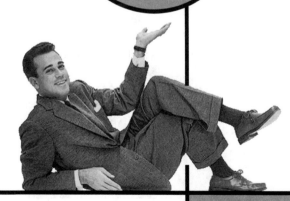

additional titles on the back!

Build Your Financial Future The Lazy Way
By Terry Meany
0-02-862648-6

Cook Your Meals The Lazy Way
By Sharon Bowers
0-02-862644-3

Organize Your Stuff The Lazy Way
By Toni Ahlgren
0-02-863000-9

Feed Your Kids Right The Lazy Way
By Virginia Van Vynckt
0-02-863001-7

Cut Your Spending The Lazy Way
By Leslie Haggin
0-02-863002-5

Stop Aging The Lazy Way
By Judy Myers, Ph.D.
0-02-862793-8

Get in Shape The Lazy Way
By Annette Cain
0-02-863010-6

Learn French The Lazy Way
By Christophe Desmaison
0-02-863011-4

Learn Italian The Lazy Way
By Gabrielle Euvino
0-02-863014-9

Learn Spanish The Lazy Way
By Steven Hawson
0-02-862650-8